SOAP
for
Internal Medicine

Look for other books in this series!

SOAP
for
Internal Medicine

Peter S. Uzelac, MD, FACOG

Series Editor
Assistant Professor
University of Southern California Keck School of Medicine
Los Angeles, California

Richard W. Moon, MD

Resident, Internal Medicine
Los Angeles County—USC Medical Center
Los Angeles, California

Angelina G. Badillo, MD

Resident, Internal Medicine
Los Angeles County—USC Medical Center
Los Angeles, California

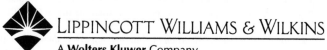

LIPPINCOTT WILLIAMS & WILKINS
A **Wolters Kluwer** Company
Philadelphia · Baltimore · New York · London
Buenos Aires · Hong Kong · Sydney · Tokyo

351 West Camden Street
Baltimore, Maryland 21201-2436 USA

530 Walnut Street
Philadelphia, Pennsylvania 19106-3621 USA

ISBN : 978-1-4051-0436-4
ISBN : 1-4051-0436-8

Library of Congress Cataloging-in-Publication Data

Uzelac, Peter S.
  SOAP for internal medicine / Peter S. Uzelac, Richard W. Moon,
  Angelina G. Badillo.
     p. ; cm.
  Includes index.
  ISBN 1-4051-0436-8 (pbk.)
  1. Medical protocols–Handbooks, manuals, etc.   2. Internal medicine–
  Handbooks, manuals, etc.
  [DNLM: 1. Internal Medicine—Handbooks]
  I. Moon, Richard W.   II. Badillo, Angelina G.   III. Title.
  RC64.U98   2005
  616–dc22

                                        2004017581

A catalogue record for this title is available from the British Library

Editor: Donna Balado
Managing Editor: Kathleen Scogna
Marketing Manager: Emilie Linkins

The publishers have made very effort to trace the copyright holders for borrowed material. If they have inadvertently overlooked any, they will be pleased to make the necessary arrangements at the first opportunity.

To purchase additional copies of this book call our customer service department at (800) 638-3030 or fax orders to (301) 824-7390. International customers should call (301) 714-2324.

Visit **Lippincott Williams & Wilkins on the Internet: http://www.lww.com**. Lippincott Williams & Wilkins customer service representatives are available from 8:30 am to 6:00 pm, EST, Monday through Friday, for telephone access.

                                                              07
                                                    4 5 6 7 8 9 10

Contents

Editors

Breck Nichols, MD, MPH
Resident, Medicine-Pediatrics
Los Angeles County-USC Medical Center
Los Angeles, California

Michael A. Polisky, MD
Resident, Medicine-Pediatrics
Los Angeles County-USC Medical Center
Los Angeles, California

Contributors

Rimma Shaposhikov, MD
Resident, Internal Medicine
Los Angeles County-USC Medical Center
Los Angeles, California

Binh Le Tran, DO
Resident, Internal Medicine
Los Angeles County-USC Medical Center
Los Angeles, California

Reviewers

Philip Carrott, Jr.
Class of 2005
The University of Kansas School of Medicine
Kansas City, Kansas

Amir A. Ghaferi
Class of 2005
The Johns Hopkins University School of Medicine
Baltimore, Maryland

Karen Moore Goldstein
Class of 2004
Duke University School of Medicine
Durham, North Carolina

Diane Lewis
Class of 2004
State University of New York Stony Brook School of Medicine
Stony Brook, New York

Syam Vasireddy, MSE
Class of 2005
University of Illinois at Chicago College of Medicine
Chicago, Illinois

To the Reader

Like most medical students, I started my ward experience head down and running, eager to finally make contact with real patients. What I found was a confusing world, completely different from anything I had known during the first two years of medical school. New language, foreign abbreviations, and residents too busy to set my bearings straight: Where would I begin?

Pocket textbooks, offering medical knowledge in a convenient and portable package, seemed to be the logical solution. Unfortunately, I found myself spending valuable time sifting through large amounts of text, often not finding the answer to my question, and in the process, missing out on teaching points during rounds!

I designed the SOAP series to provide medical students and house staff with pocket manuals that truly serve their intended purpose: quick accessibility to the most practical clinical information in a user-friendly format. At the inception of this project, I envisioned all of the benefits the SOAP format would bring to the reader:

- Learning through this model reinforces a thought process that is already familiar to students and residents, facilitating easier long-term retention.

- SOAP promotes good communication between physicians and facilitates the teaching/learning process.

- SOAP puts the emphasis back on the patient's clinical problem and not the diagnosis.

- In the age of managed care, SOAP meets the challenge of providing efficiency while maintaining quality.

- As sound medical-legal practice gains attention in physician training, SOAP emphasizes adherence to a documentation style that leaves little room for potential misinterpretation.

Rather than attempting to summarize the contents of a thousand-page textbook into a miniature form, the SOAP series focuses exclusively on guidance through patient encounters. In a typical use, "finding out where to start" or "refreshing your memory" with SOAP books should be possible in less than a minute. Subjects are always confined to two pages, and the most important points have been highlighted. Topics have been limited to those problems you will most commonly encounter repeatedly during your training, and contents are grouped according to the hospital or clinic setting. Facts and figures that are not particularly helpful to surviving life on the wards, such as demographics, pathophysiology, and busy tables and graphs, have purposely been omitted (such details are much better studied in a quiet environment using large and comprehensive texts).

Congratulations on your achievements thus far, and I wish you a highly successful medical career!

Peter S. Uzelac, MD, FACOG

Acknowledgments

I would foremost like to thank my own teachers, the physicians who have taught me their art and instilled in me the desire to pass on this knowledge to others. Special appreciation to Beverly Copland for her enthusiasm and motivation from this project's infancy, Selene Steneck for her patience and persistence in keeping this project on track, and all of the SOAP authors for their hard work and commitment to making this series a success.

Abbreviations

A-a gradient	alveolar-to-arterial gradient
Ab	antibody
Abd	abdomen
ABG	arterial blood gas
ABVD	adriamycin, bleomycin, vinblastine, and dacarbazine (regimen used to treat Hodgkin's disease)
ACE	angiotensin-converting enzyme
ACS	acute coronary syndrome
ACTH	adrenocorticotropin hormone
AD	autosomal dominant
ADH	antidiuretic hormone
AFB	acid-fast bacilli
AI	adrenal insufficiency
AIDS	acquired immunodeficiency syndrome
AIHA	autoimmune hemolytic anemia
AIN	acute interstitial nephritis
Alb	albumin
ALL	acute lymphocytic leukemia
ALT	alanine aminotransferase
AML	acute myelogenous leukemia
AMS	altered mental status
ANA	antinuclear antibody
ANCA	antineutrophil cytoplasmic antibodies
AP	alkaline phosphatase
APCR	activated protein C resistance
APL	acute promyelocytic leukemia
aPPT	activated partial thromboplastin time
AR	aortic regurgitation, autosomal recessive
ARF	acute renal failure
AS	ankylosing spondylitis, aortic stenosis
ASA	acetylsalicylic acid (aspirin)
ASD	atrial septal defect
ASMA	anti-smooth muscle antibody
AST	antimicrobial susceptibility testing
ATN	acute tubular necrosis
ATRA	all-*trans*-retinoic acid (regimen used to treat acute promyelocytic leukemia)
avF	augmented voltage foot
bid	*bis in die* (twice daily)
Bipap	bilevel positive airway pressure
BMI	body mass index
BMP	basic metabolic panel
BMT	bone marrow transplant
BP	blood pressure
bpm	beats per minute
BS	blood sugar
BUN	blood urea nitrogen

Ca	calcium
CA	cancer
CAD	coronary artery disease
c-ANCA	classic antineutrophil cytoplasmic autoantibody
Cardio	cardiovascular
CBC	complete blood count
CEA	carcinoembryonic antigen
CGD	chronic granulomatous disease
Chem7	sodium, potassium, chloride, bicarb, BUN, creatinine, glucose
CHF	congestive heart failure
CHOP	chemotherapy
CK	creatinine kinase
Cl	chloride
CLL	chronic lymphocytic leukemia
cm	centimeter
CML	chronic myelogenous leukemia
CMV	cytomegalovirus
CNS	central nervous system
COHb	carboxyhemoglobin
COPD	chronic obstructive pulmonary disease
COX	cyclooxygenase
CPDD	calcium pyrophosphate deposition disease
Cr	creatinine
CREST	calcinosis, Raynaud's disease, esophageal dysmotility, sclerodactyly, and telangiectasia
CRF	chronic renal failure
CRH	cortisol releasing hormone
CRP	C-reactive protein
CT	computed tomography
CV	cardiovascular
cx	culture
CXR	chest x-ray
D50W	50% dextrose (in water) injection
DDAVP	desmopressin acetate
DEXA	dual-energy x-ray absorptiometry
DHP	dihydropyridine
DI	diabetes insipidus
DIC	disseminated intravascular coagulation
DIP	distal interphalangeal
DKA	diabetic ketoacidosis
dL	deciliter
DM	diabetes mellitus
DNAse	deoxyribonuclease
DRE	digital rectal examination
dsDNA	double stranded DNA
DVT	deep vein thrombosis
E	ethambutol
EBV	Epstein-Barr virus
ECG	electrocardiogram
ECV	extracellular volume

EEG	electroencephalogram
EGD	esophagogastroduodenoscopy
EMG	electromyogram
ENT	ears, nose, throat
EPO	erythropoietin
ERCP	endoscopic retrograde cholangiopancreaticogram
ESR	erythrocyte sedimentation rate
ESRD	end stage renal disease
Ext	extremities
FBS	fasting blood sugar
FE_{Na}	fractional extraction of sodium
FFP	fresh frozen plasma
FHH	familial hypocalciuric hypercalcemia
FNA	fine needle aspiration
FSH	follicle-stimulating hormone
ft	feet
FUO	fever of unknown origin
g	gram
GCA	giant cell arteritis
Gen	general appearance of patient
GERD	gastroesophageal reflux disease
GFR	glomerular filtration rate
GI	gastrointestinal
GN	glomerulonephritis
GU	genitourinary
HAV	hepatitis A virus
Hb	hemoglobin
HBc	hepatitis B core
HBsAg	hepatitis B surface antigen
HBV	hepatitis B virus
HCC	hepatocellular carcinoma
HCO_3	bicarbonate
Hct	hematocrit
HCV	hepatitis C virus
HDL	high-density lipoprotein
HDV	hepatitis D virus
HEENT	head, ears, eyes, nose, throat
HEV	hepatitis E virus
Hgb	hemoglobin
HIDA	dimethyl iminodiacetic acid
HIV	human immunodeficiency virus
HL	Hodgkin's lymphoma
HONK	hyperosmolar nonketotic
H&P	history and physical
HR	heart rate
hr	hour
HRT	hormone replacement therapy
HSP	Henoch-Schönlein purpura
HSV	herpes simplex virus
Ht	height

HTN	hypertension
HUS	hemolytic uremic syndrome
I	isoniazid/INH
IBD	inflammatory bowel disease
IBM	inclusion body myositis
ICU	intensive care unit
Ig	immunoglobulin
IHSS	idiopathic hypertrophic subaortic stenosis
ILD	interstitial lung disease
IM	intramuscular
INH	isoniazid
INR	international normalized ratio
I/O	intake and output
ITP	idiopathic thrombocytopenic purpura
IU	international unit
IV	intravenous
IVDA	intravenous drug abuse
IVIG	intravenous immunoglobulin
IVP	intravenous pyelogram
JRA	juvenile rheumatoid arthritis
K	potassium
KCl	potassium chloride
kg	kilogram
KS	Kaposi's sarcoma
KUB	kidneys, ureters, bladder
L	liter
lb	pound
LDH	lactate dehydrogenase
LDL	low-density lipoprotein
LE	lower extremities
LFT	liver function test
LH	luteinizing hormone
LKM	liver-kidney microsomal antibodies
LP	lumbar puncture
LSD	lysergic acid diethylamide
MAC	mycoplasma avium complex
MAHA	macroangiopathic hemolytic anemia
mcg	microgram
MCHC	mean corpuscular hemoglobin concentration
MCP	metacarpophalangeals
MCTD	mixed connective tissue disease
MCV	mean corpuscular volume
MDRTB	multidrug resistant tuberculosis
MEN	multiple endocrine neoplasia
mEq	milliequivalent
METs	metabolic equivalents
mg	milligram
Mg	magnesium
MgO	magnesium oxide
$MgSO_4$	magnesium sulfate

MI	myocardial infarction
min	minute
mL	milliliter
mm	millimeters
mm Hg	millimeters of mercury
mmol	millimole
MOPP	mechlorethamine, vincristine, procarbazine, and prednisone
mOsm	milliosmole
MPA	medroxyprogesterone acetate
MRI	magnetic resonance imaging
MRSA	methicillin resistant *Staphylococcus aureus*
MS	mitral stenosis
MTP	metatarsophalangeal
MUGA	multiple gated acquisition
Na	sodium
NaCl	sodium chloride
NAFLD	nonalcoholic fatty liver disease
NaHCO$_3$	sodium bicarbonate
Neuro	neurologic
NH$_3$	ammonia
NHL	non-Hodgkin's lymphoma
NPH	neutral protamine Hagedorn insulin
NPO	*nulla per os* (nothing by mouth)
NS	normal saline
NSAID	nonsteroidal anti-inflammatory drug
NTG	nitroglycerin
O$_2$	oxygen
OA	osteoarthritis
OCP	oral contraceptive pill
OGTT	oral glucose tolerance test
OP	osteoporosis
O&P	ova & parasites
OR	operating room
OSA	obstructive sleep apnea
oz	ounce
PAN	polyarteritis nodosa
PaO$_2$	partial pressure of oxygen in arterial blood
PaCO$_2$	partial pressure of carbon dioxide in arterial blood
PCP	*Pneumocystis carinii* pneumonia
PE	physical examination, pulmonary embolism
PET	positron emission tomography
PFT	pulmonary function test
pH	negative log of the concentration of hydrogen
Phos	phosphorus
PIP	proximal interphalangeal
PMD	primary medical doctor
PMN	polymorphonuclear leukocytes
PMR	polymyalgia rheumatica
po	*per os* (by mouth)
pO$_2$	partial pressure of oxygen as measured by blood gas analysis

PORT	patient outcome research team
PPD	purified protein derivative
PPI	proton pump inhibitor
prn	*pro re nata* (as needed)
PSA	prostate-specific antigen
psych	psychiatric
pt	patient
PT	prothrombin time
PTH	parathyroid hormone
PTHrP	parathyroid related protein
PTT	partial thromboplastin time
PTX	pneumothorax
PUD	peptic ulcer disease
Pulm	pulmonary
PZA	pyrazinamide
q	*quodque* (every)
qh	*quaque hora* (every hour)
qd	*quaque die* (once daily)
QRS	part of ECG wave representing ventricular depolarization
R	rifampin
RA	rheumatoid arthritis
RAI	radioactive iodine
RBC	red blood cell
RDW	red cell distribution width
RF	rheumatic fever, rheumatoid factor
Rh	Rhesus factor
RI	reticulocyte index
RPR	rapid plasma reagin
RTA	renal tubular acidosis
RUQ	right upper quadrant
S	streptomycin
S_2	second heart sound
S_3	third heart sound
S_4	fourth heart sound
SaO_2	arterial oxygen concentration
sat	saturation
SBP	spontaneous bacterial peritonitis
SERMS	selective estrogen receptor modulators
SI	sacroiliac
SIADH	syndrome of inappropriate ADH
SLE	systemic lupus erythematosus
SMA	sequential multiple analyzer
s/p	status post
SQ	subcutaneous
SRP	signal recognition particle
SS	systemic sclerosis
stat	*statim* (immediately)
STD	sexually transmitted disease
TB	tuberculosis
TCA	tricyclic antidepressant

TG	triglyceride
TIBC	total iron binding capacity
tid	*ter in die* (three times daily)
TMJ	temporomandibular joint
TMP/SMX	trimethoprim/sulfamethoxazole
TMP/SMZ	trimethoprim/sulfamethoxazole
TNM	primary tumor, regional lymph nodes, and distant metastasis
TR	tricuspid regurgitation
TS	tricuspid stenosis
TSH	thyroid-stimulating hormone
TTP	thrombotic thrombocytopenic purpura
U	unit
U/A	urinalysis
μg	microgram
μl	microliter
UTI	urinary tract infection
VDRL	venereal disease research laboratory
VIP-oma	vasoactive intestinal peptide-screening tumors
VMA	vanillylmandelic acid
V/Q	ventilation-perfusion
VS	vital signs
VZV	varicella zoster virus
WBC	white blood cell
Wt	weight
x	times
y/o	years old
ZE	Zollinger-Ellison

Normal Lab Values

Blood, Plasma, Serum

Aminotransferase, alanine (ALT, SGPT)	0–35 U/L
Aminotransferase, aspartate (AST, SGOT)	0–35 U/L
Ammonia, plasma	40–80 μg/dL
Amylase, serum	0–130 U/L
Antistreptolysin O titer	Less than 150 units
Bicarbonate, serum	23–28 meq/L
Bilirubin, serum	
Total	0.3–1.2 mg/dL
Direct	0–0.3 mg/dL
Blood gases, arterial (room air)	
Po_2	80–100 mm Hg
Pco_2	35–45 mm Hg
pH	7.38–7.44
Calcium, serum	9–10.5 mg/dL
Carbon dioxide content, serum	23–28 meq/L
Chloride, serum	98–106 meq/L
Cholesterol, total, plasma	150–199 mg/dL (desirable)
Cholesterol, low-density lipoprotein (LDL), plasma	$\leq$ 130 mg/dL (desirable)
Cholesterol, high-density lipoprotein (HDL), plasma	$\geq$ 40 mg/dL (desirable)
Complement, serum	
C3	55–120 mg/dL
Total	37–55 U/mL
Copper, serum	70–155 μg/dL
Creatine kinase, serum	30–170 U/L
Creatinine, serum	0.7–1.3 mg/dL
Ethanol, blood	< 50 mg/dL
Fibrinogen, plasma	150–350 mg/dL
Folate, red cell	160–855 ng/mL
Folate, serum	2.5–20 ng/mL
Glucose, plasma	
Fasting	70–105 mg/dL
2 hours postprandial	< 140 mg/dL
Iron, serum	60–160 μg/dL
Iron-binding capacity, serum	250–460 μg/dL
Lactate dehydrogenase, serum	60–100 U/L
Lactic acid, venous blood	6–16 mg/dL
Lead, blood	< 40 μg/dL

Lipase, serum	< 95 U/L
Magnesium, serum	1.5–2.4 mg/dL
Manganese, serum	0.3–0.9 ng/mL
Methylmalonic acid, serum	150–370 nmol/L
Osmolality plasma	275–295 mOsm/kg H_2O
Phosphatase, acid, serum	0.5–5.5 U/L
Phosphatase, alkaline, serum	36–92 U/L
Phosphorus, inorganic, serum	3–4.5 mg/dL
Potassium, serum	3.5–5 meq/L
Protein, serum	
Total	6.0–7.8 g/dL
Albumin	3.5–5.5 g/dL
Globulins	2.5–3.5 g/dL
Alpha$_1$	0.2–0.4 g/dL
Alpha$_2$	0.5–0.9 g/dL
Beta	0.6–1.1 g/dL
Gamma	0.7–1.7 g/dL
Rheumatoid factor	< 40 U/mL
Sodium, serum	136–145 meq/L
Triglycerides	< 150 mg/dL (desirable)
Urea nitrogen, serum	8–20 mg/dL
Uric acid, serum	2.5–8 mg/dL
Vitamin B_{12}, serum	200–800 pg/mL

Cerebrospinal Fluid

Cell count	0–5 cells/μL
Glucose (less than 40% of simultaneous plasma concentration is abnormal)	40–80 mg/dL
Protein	15–60 mg/dL
Pressure (opening)	70–200 cm H_2O

Endocrine

Adrenocorticotropin (ACTH)	9–52 pg/mL
Aldosterone, serum	
Supine	2–5 ng/dL
Standing	7–20 ng/dL
Aldosterone, urine	5–19 μg/24 h
Cortisol	
Serum 8 AM	8–20 μg/dL
5 PM	3–13 μg/dL

1 h after cosyntropin	> 18 μg/dL
usually ≥ 8 μg/dL above baseline	
overnight suppression test	< 5 μg/dL
Urine free cortisol	< 90 μg/24 h
Estradiol, serum	
Male	10–30 pg/mL
Female	
Cycle day 1–10	50–100 pmol/L
Cycle day 11–20	50–200 pmol/L
Cycle day 21–30	70–150 pmol/L
Estriol, urine	> 12 mg/24 h
Follicle-stimulating hormone, serum	
Male (adult)	5–15 mU/mL
Female	
Follicular or luteal phase	5–20 mU/mL
Midcycle peak	30–50 mU/mL
Postmenopausal	> 35 mU/mL
Insulin, serum (fasting)	5–20 mU/L
17-ketosteroids, urine	
Male	8–22 mg/24 h
Female	Up to 15 μg/24 h
Luteinizing hormone, serum	
Male	3–15 mU/mL (3–15 U/L)
Female	
Follicular or luteal phase	5–22 mU/mL
Midcycle peak	30–250 mU/mL
Postmenopausal	> 30 mU/mL
Parathyroid hormone, serum	10–65 pg/mL
Progesterone	
Luteal	3–30 ng/mL
Follicular	< 1 ng/mL
Prolactin, serum	
Male	< 15 ng/mL
Female	< 20 ng/mL
Testosterone, serum	
Adult male	300–1200 ng/dL
Female	20–75 ng/dL
Thyroid function tests (normal ranges vary)	
Thyroid iodine (^{131}I) uptake	10% to 30% of administered dose at 24 h

Thyroid-stimulating hormone (TSH)	0.5–5.0 μU/mL
Thyroxine (T4), serum	
Total	5–12 pg/dL
Free	0.9–2.4 ng/dL
Free T4 index	4–11
Triiodothyronine, resin (T3)	25%–35%
Triiodothyronine, serum (T3)	70–195 ng/dL
Vitamin D	
1,25-dihydroxy, serum	25–65 pg/mL
25-hydroxy, serum	15–80 ng/mL

Gastrointestinal

Fecal urobilinogen	40–280 mg/24 h
Gastrin, serum	0–180 pg/mL
Lactose tolerance test	
Increase in plasma glucose	> 15 mg/dL
Lipase, ascitic fluid	< 200 U/L
Secretin-cholecystokinin pancreatic function	> 80 meq/L of HCO_3 in at least 1 specimen collected over 1 h
Stool fat	< 5 g/d on a 100-g fat diet
Stool nitrogen	< 2 g/d
Stool weight	< 200 g/d

Hematology

Activated partial thromboplastin time	25–35 s
Bleeding time	< 10 min
Coagulation factors, plasma	
Factor I	150–350 mg/dL
Factor II	60%–150% of normal
Factor V	60%–150% of normal
Factor VII	60%–150% of normal
Factor VIII	60%–150% of normal
Factor IX	60%–150% of normal
Factor X	60%–150% of normal
Factor XI	60%–150% of normal
Factor XII	60%–150% of normal
Erythrocyte count	4.2–5.9 million cells/μL
Erythropoietin	< 30 mU/mL
D-dimer	< 0.5 μg/mL

Ferritin, serum	15–200 ng/mL
Glucose-6-phosphate dehydrogenase, blood	5–15 U/g Hgb
Haptoglobin, serum	50–150 mg/dL
Hematocrit	
Male	41%–51%
Female	36%–47%
Hemoglobin, blood	
Male	14–17 g/dL
Female	12–16 g/dL
Hemoglobin, plasma	0.5–5 mg/dL
Leukocyte alkaline phosphatase	15–40 mg of phosphorus liberated/h per 10^{10} cells
Score	13–130/100 polymorphonuclear neutrophils and band forms
Leukocyte count	
Nonblacks	4000–10,000/μL
Blacks	3500–10,000/μL
Lymphocytes	
CD4+ cell count	640–1175/μL
CD8+ cell count	335–875/μL
CD4 : CD8 ratio	1.0–4.0
Mean corpuscular hemoglobin (MCH)	28–32 pg
Mean corpuscular hemoglobin concentration (MCHC)	32–36 g/dL
Mean corpuscular volume (MCV)	80–100 fL
Platelet count	150,000–350,000/μL
Protein C activity, plasma	67%–I 31%
Protein C resistance	2.2–2.6
Protein S activity, plasma	82%–144%
Prothrombin time	11–13 s
Reticulocyte count	0.5%–1.5% of erythrocytes
Absolute	23,000–90,000 cells/μL
Schilling test (oral administration of radioactive cobalamin-labeled vitamin B_{12})	8.5%–28% excreted in urine per 24–48 h
Sedimentation rate, erythrocyte (Westergren)	
Male	0–15 mm/h
Female	0–20 mm/h

Volume, blood
  Plasma
    Male   25–44 mL/kg body weight
    Female   28–43 mL/kg body weight
  Erythrocyte
    Male   25–35 mL/kg body weight
    Female   20–30 mL/kg body weight

Urine

Amino acids	200–400 mg/24 h
Amylase	6.5–48.1 U/h
Calcium	100–300 mg/d on unrestricted diet
Chloride	80–250 meq/d (varies with intake)
Copper	0–100 μg/24 h
Creatine	
Male	4–40 mg/24 h
Female	0–100 mg/24 h
Creatinine	15–25 mg/kg per 24 h
Creatinine clearance	90–140 mL/min
Osmolality	38–1400 mOsm/kg H_2O
Phosphate, tubular resorption	79%–94% (0.79–0.94) of filtered load
Potassium	25–100 meq/24 h (varies with intake)
Protein	< 100 mg/24 h
Sodium	100–260 meq/24 h (varies with intake)
Uric acid	250–750 mg/24 h (varies with diet)
Urobilinogen	0.05–2.5 mg/24 h

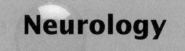

I

Neurology

S What is the headache like?

Certain symptoms should raise immediate red flags, such as sudden onset that feels like "the worst headache of my life" should make you think of subarachnoid hemorrhage.

Band-like sensations are seen in tension headaches.

Consistent, brief, severe, nonpulsatile headaches (30 to 60 min) in older men are often seen in cluster headaches.

Severe, pulsatile headaches, involving usually one side of the head but occasionally both, associated with photophobia, phonophobia, nausea, and vomiting, are likely to be migraines.

- Pts will usually state that they prefer to lie down in a dark room.

Ask about associated symptoms

Fever: seen in meningitis

Photophobia: meningitis or migraine headache

Nausea, vomiting, with or without auras: migraine headache

Arthralgias and pain over temples: temporal arteritis

Personality changes: intracranial mass

Purulent nasal discharge: sinusitis

Take a good medical history, focusing on the following

Hypertension: hypertensive encephalopathy

Medications: atenolol, digoxin, nitroglycerin, H_2 blockers

- *Anticoagulation*: Intracranial hemorrhage can occur in severely elevated international normalized ratio.

History of trauma: epidural hematoma

History of cancer: Think about brain metastases, which may also bleed.

Immunocompromised: atypical and bacterial meningitis, toxoplasmosis

O Perform a thorough PE, looking for the following signs

Fever: seen in meningitis

Blood pressure: Severe hypertension could herald hypertensive emergency, stroke, or bleed.

Papilledema: increased intracranial pressure

Dental caries: dental abscess, caries, or gingivitis

Neck flexion–associated pain: Suggests meningeal irritation, which can occur with meningitis or subarachnoid hemorrhage.

Petechial rash on lower extremities: meningococcal meningitis

Neurologic deficit or focal weakness: ischemic or hemorrhagic stroke

Sinus tenderness to palpation: sinusitis

Tight, cord-like tender temporal artery: rare but sometimes associated with temporal arteritis

Temporomandibular joint: Jaw clicks with mouth opening and closing, causing pain.

Ears: Otitis media or externa can also cause pain. Otitis externa in a diabetic is an ENT emergency.

A Headache

When thinking about a headache, remember what can cause pain in the head:

- *External musculature*: Most common, causing a band-like sensation when tension occurs in a tension headache.

- *Sinuses*: When inflamed with pressure exerted from within, pain can result from sinusitis.
- *Jaw*: Both caries/dental abscesses and temporomandibular joint problems can radiate pain throughout the head.
- *Ears*: Pain can radiate into head.
- *Nerves*: Neural inflammation is a rare cause of pain. If pt has burning sensation on one side of his or her face, it is possible that he or she has trigeminal neuralgia.
- *Vasculature*: Vasodilation or constriction can cause pain. While the pathophysiology of migraine is not yet fully understood, it is thought that these headaches occur when the cerebral arteries dilate rapidly after being constricted. Arterial inflammation can also produce pain in the case of temporal arteritis.
- *Meninges*: Meningeal inflammation (meningitis) or irritation with blood (subarachnoid hemorrhage) can produce severe pain.

Remember that there are no pain sensory fibers within the brain. Cerebrovascular ischemic and hemorrhagic events rarely produce pain.

Rule out life-threatening causes first

- Subdural hematoma	- Epidural hematoma
- Subarachnoid hemorrhage	- Ischemic or hemorrhagic stroke
- Hypertensive encephalopathy	- Intracranial mass
- Temporal arteritis	- Meningitis

Once you have ruled out these serious causes of headaches, the remaining diagnoses are most likely either sinusitis, tension headache, cluster headache, or migraine headache

P

Consider a stat head CT
Only if there is clinical suspicion of stroke, mass, or bleed

Consider lumbar puncture if CT is negative with no evidence of increased intracranial pressure and there is clinical suspicion of meningitis, subarachnoid hemorrhage, or altered mental status
Bacterial meningitis: elevated PMNs, low glucose, elevated protein, positive cerebrospinal fluid (CSF) culture, CSF to blood glucose ratio < 0.4
Intracranial bleeds: numerous RBCs, increased PMNs, increased protein ($\sim$ 1 mg protein per 1000 RBCs)
Traumatic taps vs. intracranial bleeds: In traumatic taps, the amount of RBCs tapers off from the 1st tube to the last tube, whereas in intracranial bleeds it does not.

Treat the underlying cause
Mass lesion, intracranial bleed: neurosurgery consult
Ischemia: see Cardiology section, p. 29–47
Meningitis: 3rd-generation cephalosporin +/− dexamethasone
Encephalitis: Acyclovir because herpes simplex virus is sometimes the etiology
Temporal arteritis: Start prednisone and call an ENT specialist for a temporal artery biopsy.
Sinusitis: amoxicillin with clavulanate for 14 to 21 days
Tension headache: acetaminophen, NSAIDs
Cluster headache: NSAIDs, ergotamine, sumatriptan, inhaled oxygen
Migraine headache: aspirin, acetaminophen, NSAIDs, ergotamine, sumatriptan

S **Ask the family, witnesses, or the pt if the onset was sudden**
It is important to distinguish between delirium and dementia, the two major classes of altered mental status (AMS):
- *Delirium*: sudden onset over hrs to days
- *Dementia*: insidious onset over wks to months

Has the pt had any memory loss, difficulty with activities of daily living (e.g., cooking, finances), missing appointments, and inaccurate or inappropriate answers to questions?
This constellation of symptoms usually points to dementia.

Does the pt have any conditions that are potential causes for delirium?
Drugs: cocaine, opiates, benzodiazepines, antihistamines
Tumor: primary brain tumor, metastatic brain tumor
Nutrition: vitamin B_{12} deficiency, folate deficiency
Ischemia: cerebrovascular disease
Infections: syphilis, meningitis, sepsis, HIV
Alcohol: intoxication, withdrawal, hepatic encephalopathy
Trauma: subdural hematoma, epidural hematoma, parenchymal bleed
Metabolic: hyperglycemia, hypoglycemia, uremia, hypernatremia, hyponatremia, hypercalcemia
Pulm: hypercapnia, hypoxia
Endocrine: hypothyroidism, hyperthyroidism
Vasculitic: systemic lupus erythematosus, rheumatoid arthritis, other vasculitides

O **Perform a focused PE, looking for red flags for reversible causes of AMS**
Fever may indicate meningitis, but it could also indicate a cerebral vasculitis or TTP.
Dry skin, lateral thinning of eyebrows, and wiry hair are hallmark signs of hypothyroidism, which can cause myxedema coma.
Sweaty skin, intense stare, rapid heart rate, and thin frame are the common presenting symptoms of hyperthyroidism, which can lead to thyroid storm, in which pts can be altered with or without fever. This is an endocrinologic emergency.
Neurologic deficits suggest stroke.

Perform a Folstein mini-mental status exam
The mini-mental status is a test with a score out of 30 possible points. A score less than 25 indicates significant mental deficit.
Sudden alterations in orientation suggest delirium.
Deficits in memory and cognitive abilities suggest dementia.

A **Altered Mental Status**
Delirium occurs when a medical condition causes the pt's alteration in mental status.
Dementia occurs secondary to progressive destruction of the brain tissue and is often
(but not always) associated with aging.

Differential diagnosis
Delirium:
- Drugs
- Ischemic encephalopathies
- Trauma
- Medications
- Infections
- Tumor
- Metabolic
  encephalopathies
- Vasculitis
- Endocrine

Dementia:
- Multi-infarct dementia
  (vascular)
- Alzheimer's disease
- Lewy body type

If you are confident that your pt has none of the above conditions, consider that the pt
may be experiencing psychosis.

P **Obtain following laboratories for all pts with AMS**
- CBC
- BUN, creatinine,
  glucose
- Calcium
- Urinalysis
- Vitamin B_{12}
- TSH
- PT, aPTT
- ABG
- Liver transaminases
- Folate
- Electrolyte panel
- RPR, VDRL
- Troponin
- Urine, serum toxicology
- ESR

If clinically warranted, consider ordering the following studies
- Stat head CT
- Chest x-ray
- Lumbar puncture
- ECG

If you suspect chronic alcoholism or malnourishment, consider empirically treating with 100 mg of thiamine IV first, followed by one ampule of 50% dextrose
To prevent Wernicke-Korsakoff syndrome.

If you suspect an overdose of opiates or benzodiazepines, consider empirically treating with the following
Naloxone for narcotic or opiate overdose
Flumazenil for benzodiazepine overdose

For pts who are altered and agitated, you may use Haldol 5 mg IM
This antipsychotic medication can be very effective in delirious pts.

If the pt is definitely delirious, consider maintaining light in the pt's room and keep a large, updated calendar and clock on the wall
This will reorient the pt and help prevent sundowning (an episode of peculiar behavior
that occurs during worsening of delirium at night).

For pts with dementia, consider starting a cholinesterase inhibitor and discuss with the pt's family regarding chronic care
It is always important to broach these topics with the family earlier than later.

If all of the above laboratory tests are negative, a psychiatry consult is indicated

S **Does the pt report a loss of consciousness?**
By definition, syncope is a transient loss of consciousness.
Pts may confuse the following conditions that do not involve loss of consciousness:
- Vertigo   - Presyncope   - Lightheadedness

Does the pt report any symptoms before loss of consciousness?
A detailed account of symptoms before, during, or after episode may reveal underlying mechanism:
- Palpitations suggest cardiac etiology such as arrhythmias.
- Changes in position suggest orthostatic hypotension.
- Pallor, diaphoresis, and lightheadedness suggest neurally mediated.

Does the pt report any precipitating factors?
Wearing tight collars or shaving suggest carotid sinus.
Exercise or exertional factors
Emotional events or stress

Does pt give history of a seizure disorder?
Seizures are difficult to distinguish from syncope.
Seizures may involve auras or disorientation after the event.

Were there any witnesses?
Witnesses of the episode may report seizure activity or other details of the event.

Review medications
Take a detailed drug history, include recent changes or additions.
Orthostatic hypotension is a common side effect of many drugs, such as:
- Diruetics
- ACE inhibitors
- Nitrates

Arrhythmias: β-blockers, digoxin, antiarrhythmics, tricyclic antidepressants

Does the pt report a family history with similar or cardiac symptoms?
Cardiac disease: Family members who died of sudden death may indicate prolonged QT syndrome or Wolff-Parkinson-White syndrome.
Psychiatric illness

O **Review vital signs**
If positive orthostatics, consider medications vs. volume contraction.
Measure blood pressure in both arms.
Hemodynamic instability is suggested by tachycardia, hypotension.

Perform PE
Gen: assess level of consciousness (postictal?)
HEENT: presence of bruit
Heart: irregular rate, murmurs, displaced point of maximal impulse, jugular venous pressure
Neuro: focal deficits

Review the results of the CBC
Anemia may worsen orthostasis.

Check the comprehensive metabolic panel
Increased BUN/Cr (volume contraction) puts pt at risk for orthostatic hypotension.
Electrolyte abnormalities rarely cause loss of consciousness.

Consider urine toxicology screen
Consider intoxication as possible cause.

Consider ABG
Calculate A-a gradient; if elevated, consider pulmonary embolus (PE).

Consider pregnancy test in women of childbearing age
With nearly any complaint, consider pregnancy in women of childbearing age.

Consider ECG
Not diagnostic but may be helpful if Wolff-Parkinson-White syndrome, Brugada, or arrhythmia.

Consider CXR
To assess cardiac size if cardiac disease is suspected.

 Syncope
Transient loss of consciousness

Etiologies
- Neurally mediated (vasovagal)
- Psychiatric
- Neurologic disease
- Cardiac-mediated: aortic stenosis, arrhythmia
- Medications
- Unknown
- Carotid sinus syndrome
- Orthostatic hypotension
- Subclavian steal syndrome

Differential diagnosis
- Seizure
- PE
- Tamponade
- Arteriovenous malformation
- Intoxication
- Stroke
- Hypoglycemia
- Hypothermia
- Pneumothorax
- Hypotension
- Panic attack
- Hypoxia
- Internal bleed
- Electrolyte abnormalities
- Migraine

P **Admit pts with any of the following for monitoring**
Structural heart disease (congestive heart failure, coronary artery disease, valvular disease)
- Suspect ischemia or arrhythmias
- Severe orthostatics
- Abnormal ECG
- Suspect cerebrovascular accident

Perform further diagnostic workup if cardiac etiology is suspected
Assess left ventricular function or valvular disease with stress testing or echocardiography to rule out ischemia.
Arrhythmias can be tested by Holter, continuous loop monitoring, or electrophysiologic studies.
Rule out myocardial infarction with serial troponins and ECG.

If you suspect orthostatic hypotension, address volume status
Discontinue any offending medications.
Volume replacement
Fluorocortisone (autonomic failure)

If you suspect neurocardiogenic-mediated etiology in a pt with normal ECG and no evidence of heart disease, obtain tilt table testing
Make sure that pts with risk factors for cardiovascular disease have a stress test first.

If you suspect neurologic disease, consider CT head or EEG
Useful to help rule out seizure and intracranial bleed or mass.

If you suspect psychiatric etiology and previous etiologies have been ruled out, consult psychiatry

S **Are there any focal neurologic symptoms?**
Stroke often presents with hemiparesis, aphasia, dysarthria, sensory loss, or a sudden
   change in cognitive function.
Pts may present with generalized symptoms such as stupor, seizures, delirium, or coma.

When was the onset of the neurologic symptoms?
If not known, when was the last known time that neurologic function was intact. This
   question is *crucial*. In addition to providing important information about onset, this
   will help determine if ischemic stroke pts are eligible for thrombolytic therapy.

**Review the pt's history for risk factors for ischemic
or hemorrhagic stroke**
As you begin working up a pt for stroke, it is paramount to distinguish whether the pt
   falls into one category or the other because the treatments are vastly different.
Risk factors for ischemic stroke include:
                - Atrial fibrillation   - Transient ischemic attack or prior ischemic stroke
                - Carotid disease   - Hypercoagulable state   - Coronary artery disease
                - Diabetes
Risk factors for hemorrhagic stroke include:
                - Uncontrolled hypertension   - Trauma   - Fall

O **Conduct a focused PE, concentrating on the neurologic exam**
Certain strokes and affected vessels can present in a certain pattern:
   - *Lacunar*: pure motor or pure sensory deficit, contralateral to affected side with
     ipsilateral ataxia, dysarthria, crural paresis
   - *Middle cerebral artery*: contralateral hemiplegia, sensory loss, global aphasia, and
     homonymous hemianopsia
   - *Anterior cerebral artery*: contralateral paresis of lower extremity and sensory loss,
     rigidity, urinary incontinence, delirium
   - *Cerebellar artery*: contralateral spinothalamic tract loss, vertigo, nausea/vomiting,
     nystagmus, ipsilateral limb ataxia

Obtain and review emergent head CT without IV contrast
Although ischemic changes are not best visualized in this modality (frequently
   appearing normal in earlier phases), CT scan is effective at visualizing fresh blood.
   This is an excellent way of rapidly ascertaining if a hemorrhagic stroke has occurred.
It may also show masses, fractures, or evidence of increased intracranial pressure.
CT is also usually more readily available and can be obtained more quickly than MRI.

Perform lumbar puncture in pts with normal head CT
Rule out meningitis and can possibly reveal occult subarachnoid hemorrhage.

Laboratory workup
            - CBC   - Chem 7   - PT/PTT   - Troponin
            - Liver function   - Blood cultures - RPR/VDRL

Conduct imaging workup, as well
            - Chest x-ray   - ECG   - Carotid ultrasound
            - EEG   - Echocardiogram   - MRI

Stroke, sometimes referred to as a cerebrovascular accident
No tissue is more dependent on a constant supply of oxygen and glucose than central nervous tissue. Metabolic failure occurs within 10 seconds of blood flow stoppage. Within minutes, neuronal injury occurs. Even then function can be recovered, but after that time tissue begins to die. Once tissue dies, brain edema begins to occur, and the mass effect from this can further impair neuronal recovery. There are three types of clinical manifestations of stroke:
- *Transient ischemic attack*: Symptoms resolve completely within 24 hrs.
- *Reversible ischemic neurologic deficit*: Symptoms resolve completely within 1 wk.
- *Complete stroke*: Complete recovery never occurs.

Be sure to further classify the stroke based on available findings
Ischemic
- Lacunar	- Cerebellar	- Anterior cerebral artery
- Middle cerebral artery	- Vertebrobasilar	

Hemorrhagic
- Often there will be evolving/changing physical symptoms as the hemorrhagic area grows or stabilizes.

 Protect the pt in the initial moments
Provide oxygen and assess the need for intubation for any pt with altered mental status.
If hemorrhagic stroke has been ruled out, consider deep venous thrombosis prophylaxis.

Monitor blood pressure
If diastolic blood pressure is greater than 140 mm Hg, start nitroprusside IV drip to slowly reduce blood pressure over the next 36 to 48 hrs to normal.
In this case, higher blood pressures than normal can be tolerated to improve cerebral perfussion pressure.
Avoid rapid blood pressure reduction, which can exacerbate existing ischemic stroke.

Give thrombolytics in pts with suspected ischemic stroke and without evidence of hemorrhagic stroke
Tissue plasminogen activator is commonly used.
- *Indications*: Pts are at least 18 years old, with clinically significant neurologic evidence of ischemic stroke, AND less than 3 hrs since last known normal neurologic state.
- *Contraindications*:
- Intracranial bleed	- Active internal bleeding
- Coagulopathy	- Severe hypertension out of control
- Recent lumbar puncture	- Rapidly improving symptoms
- History of gastrointestinal or genitourinary bleeding in last 3 wks	

Follow up treated pts
Check for bleeding
No heparin, warfarin, or aspirin for first 24 hrs

For pts with hemorrhagic stroke
Avoid heparin, tissue plasminogen activator, and antiplatelet drugs.
Target systolic blood pressure of 140–160 mm Hg. Obtain neurosurgical consult.

After pt is stabilized, image with MRI and institute physical and occupational therapy

S

What were the pt's symptoms (ask pt, family, or witnesses)?
Primary generalized seizures have a symmetric bilateral onset.
- *Tonic-clonic seizures* begin with a tonic phase and are followed by alternating movements that characterize the clonic phase.
- *Absence seizures*, more common in pediatric populations, present with a brief loss of consciousness and eye blinking.

Partial seizures have a focal onset.
- *Simple partial seizures* have preserved consciousness with focal motor or sensory symptoms (one part of the body or face). These can often be preceded by olfactory, gustatory, bizarre sensory symptoms, which is part of the aura phenomenon.
- *Complex partial seizures* arise commonly from the temporal lobe and are characterized by loss of consciousness, lip smacking, lack of focal motor activity, and a state of delirium or stupor. Often, secondary generalization may occur.

Is there any past medical history that can cause seizures?
- Alcohol or drug withdrawal   - Meningitis   - Liver failure
- Cerebrovascular disease   - Space-occupying lesions (such as malignancy)

What medicines is the pt taking?
- Ciprofloxacin   - Cyclosporine   - Cyclophosphamide
- Lidocaine   - Imipenem   - Penicillin
- Isoniazid   - Tricyclic antidepressants

If pt is taking antiepileptic medication for a past history of seizures, note the dosage and frequency, recent changes in doses, and compliance with these medicines.

O

Review vital signs
Greatest concern often surrounds airway management during and after the seizure, so respiratory rate and oxygen saturation are therefore of paramount importance.
Fever may indicate an infectious process, either intracranial (meningitis, encephalitis) or extracranial (shigella).

Perform PE
Concentrate on the motor symptoms to characterize the seizures.
- *Neuro exam*: responsiveness, pupillary reaction, reflexes, posture, tone
- *Seizure stopped*: responsive and verbally communicates and follows commands
- *Seizure ongoing*: tachycardia, eye deviation, increased tone, and/or clonic movements

Review laboratory tests
Seizures can present with disorders of blood glucose, serum sodium, calcium, magnesium phosphate, ammonia, and BUN/creatinine.
CBC (anemia) and ABG (hypoxia) are also important causes of seizure to note.
Check troponin levels, urine toxicology, and consider cultures of blood, sputum, and urine if the pt has a fever (infection).
Antiepileptic drug levels (phenytoin, phenobarbital) are also important to note.

Obtain relevant imaging studies
Chest x-ray: This will look for an aspiration that may have occurred during the seizure.
CT head without contrast: Rule out hemorrhage, hydrocephalus, or space-occupying lesion.
MRI brain: Greater sensitivity for ischemia, infarction, and space-occupying lesions.

Obtain lumbar puncture in pts with normal head CT
This will help rule out encephalitis or meningitis.

Obtain an EEG
This will confirm seizure activity, even if the pt may not physically manifest signs of a seizure while under heavy sedation.

Seizure
Seizure represents a massive neuronal discharge in the brain manifesting as physical symptoms.

Note the type of seizure based on available information (e.g., generalized tonic-clonic, absence, simple partial, or complex partial).

Differential diagnosis
Myoclonus: brief muscle contraction that is shock-like
  • Can be seen with cardiac resuscitative efforts.

Dystonia: sustained muscle contraction (such as torticollis) that can be a result of drug reactions (metoclopramide, haloperidol)

Begin by stabilizing the pt. This includes managing the oral airway, administering oxygen, and giving thiamine 100 mg IV followed by dextrose 50 g IV once
Additional seizure precautions include keeping the bedrails (preferably padded) up at all times and rotating the pt over to his or her left side to prevent aspiration.

Give a benzodiazepine
Lorazepam 2 mg IV: Repeat every 5 to 10 min up to a total of 8 mg or until the seizure stops.
  • This is especially useful for pts who have alcohol-related seizure.
  • Be sure to monitor the pt for decreases in respiratory rate and blood pressure.

Treat or correct the underlying disorders
| - Infections | - Liver failure | - Hypoglycemia |
| - Hypernatremia | - Hyponatremia | - Renal failure |

Also discontinue all medicines that can induce seizures unless essential.

Then, provide phenytoin as acute or chronic therapy of seizures
Load 15 mg/kg IV at a maximum rate of 50 mg/min.

Watch for ataxia, nystagmus, nausea, vomiting, and diplopia, all common side effects.

Afterward, daily therapy consists of 5 mg/kg/day IV or po divided bid or tid.

Check levels regularly.

For refractory seizures, give phenobarbital
Load 10 mg/kg IV no faster than 50 mg/min.

Again observe the pt for sedation and decreased respiratory rate.

The pt can be maintained on many other medications as an outpatient, including valproic acid, carbamazepine, gabapentin, topiramate, and lamotrigene
For assistance with starting these medications, consult a neurologist.

S **Is there an exaggerated sense of motion or motion when there is no motion at all?**

These are classic symptoms of vertigo.

It is crucial to distinguish this from syncope, light-headedness, or imbalance, which do not suggest a vestibular origin.

Is the onset sudden? Is it associated with nausea, vomiting, difficulty walking or standing, tinnitus, or hearing loss?

A "yes" answer to these questions strongly suggests a peripheral vestibulopathy.

Have the symptoms developed gradually?

These symptoms are more typical of a central lesion.

How long do the episodes last? Are there auditory symptoms present?

Table 1 will help classify common causes of vertigo based on history.

O **Perform a focused neurologic exam**

Gait evaluation, including Romberg test

- *Fukuda test*: Walk in place, eyes closed, rotating to affected/diseased labyrinthe.

Nystagmus

- Horizontal with rotatory component; fast phase beats away from affected side in peripheral vestibulopathy. These are usually suppressed by visual fixation.
- Vertical nystagmus, nonfatigable, and unsuppressed by visual fixation suggests central lesion.
- Nystagmus can be induced by positions termed the Nylen-Barany maneuvers (moving from sitting position with head turned to side, quickly placed supine with head 30 degrees lower than body; repeat with head turned to left and again, looking straight)

Consider further workup as needed to distinguish central from peripheral lesions:

      - Audiologic evaluation   - Caloric stimulation

      - MRI scan   - Electronystagmography

A **Vertigo**

Comment whether you feel the lesion is central or peripherally based.

Table 1 Common Causes of Vertigo by Symptom		
Duration of Vertigo	**(+) Auditory Symptoms**	**(−) Auditory Symptoms**
Seconds	Perilymphatic fistula	Positional vertigo Vertebrobasilar insufficiency Cervical vertigo
Hours	Meniere disease Syphillis	Recurrent vestibulopathy Vestibular migraine
Days	Labyrinthitis	Vestibular neuronitis
Months	Acoustic neuroma Ototoxicity	Multiple sclerosis Cerebellar degeneration

Possible peripheral causes include
Meniere disease (endolymphatic hydrops): a disease of unknown etiology with the triad
  of vertigo, tinnitus, and decreased hearing on the affected side.
  • It is chronic with few effective therapies.
Labrythinitis: inflammation (usually caused by viral infection) of the vestibular system.
  Also known as *otitis interna.*
  • Self-limited disease
Positional vertigo: a benign condition in which vertigo occurs with certain head
  movements
Vestibular neuronitits: inflammation of the vestibular component of the eighth cranial
  nerve
  • Usually viral, most likely herpetic
Acoustic neuroma/Schwannoma: tumor of the eighth cranial nerve
Traumatic vertigo: Can be just like labyrinthitis, but there is a traumatic onset.
Perilymphatic fistula: endolymph draining into the middle ear

Possible central causes
Brainstem: ischemia or tumor of the medulla at the location of the vestibular nucleus.
Cerebellar tumors
Multiple sclerosis: immune-mediated destruction of white matter can lead to vertigo if
  in the correct location.

Differential diagnosis
Medications can simulate vertigo:

- Anticonvulsants	- Antibiotics	- Hypnotics
- Analgesics	- Alcohol	- Sedatives

Psychogenic vertigo: associated with anxiety disorders; nystagmus will not be present.

P **Treat according to working diagnosis. For any diagnosis, consider
consulting an otolaryngologic specialist to evaluate the pt**
Positional vertigo
Frequent positional change to reposition otoconia in semicircular canals. These are
  called Dix-Hallpike maneuvers.

Meniere disease
Start pt on a low-salt diet and diuretics. Therapy is rarely effective.

Perilymphatic fistula
Consider surgical repair.

Provide general symptomatic relief from vertiginous episodes
Bed rest for acute vertigo; exercise for chronic vertigo to increase tolerance
Antihistamines, anticholinergics
Sedatives, such as diazepam, with antiemetic for severe acute vertigo attack
Scopolamine
Meclizine
Physical therapy
Consider prednisone if other medical management fails.
Aminoglycosides can cause selective chemical destruction of vestibular hair cell, so they
  should be avoided.
Also consider selective surgical section of vestibular portion of eighth cranial nerve or
  labyrinthectomy.

II

Pulmonary

S **What are the pt's symptoms?**
- Fever
- Blood-streaked sputum
- Cough with or without purulent sputum
- Dyspnea

When was the onset of symptoms?

Strictly defined, symptoms of community-acquired pneumonia begin outside the hospital.
- If symptoms begin in the hospital, they must begin within 48 hrs to be considered community acquired.
- If greater than 48 hrs since admission, or if pt usually resides in a long-term facility, the possibility of nosocomial pneumonia must be considered.

What are the pt's age, gender, and comorbidities?

All of these factors determine points in the PORT classification system (see following):
- Male gender is a risk in pneumonia and thus females receive minus 10 points.
- Age in years equals a number of points.
- Nursing home residence also contributes 10 points.
- Comorbidities also have point values: nondermatologic neoplasias (30 points), liver disease (20 points), congestive heart failure (CHF, 10 points), renal disease (10 points), and cerebrovascular disease (10 points).

Is there any history of recent aspiration?
If so, consider the presence of anaerobic or polymicrobial organisms; choose broader antibiotics.

Does the pt seem able to comply with outpatient antibiotic therapy?
Inability to comply with empiric therapy would mandate hospital admission.

O **Review vital signs**
These provide an idea of the severity of disease.
The following are associated with greater morbidity:
- Temperature greater than 40° C or less than 35° C (15 points)
- Heart rate > 125 beats per minute (10 points)
- Respiratory rate > 30 breaths per minute (20 points)
- Systolic blood pressure < 90 mm Hg (20 points)
- Altered mental status (20 points)

Perform a thorough pulmonary examination
Bronchial breath sounds, rales, and dullness to percussion are common findings.

Obtain a CBC, Chem 7, CXR, and ABG
Certain values will register points toward the PORT risk classification score:
- Hct < 30% (10 points)
- Sodium < 130 meq/L (20 points)
- Arterial pH < 7.35 (30 points)
- Pleural effusion (10 points)
- BUN > 30 mg/dL (20 points)
- Glucose > 250 mg/dL (10 points)
- pO_2 of > 60 mm Hg (10 points)

Other values of note would be increased WBC count with a bandemia ("left shift") and an acidosis, either respiratory or metabolic.
CXR often will show one or more areas of lobar consolidations with air bronchograms.

Obtain a sputum sample for Gram stain and culture before administering antibiotics
Some argue that the findings will have poor positive and negative predictive values, but the Gram stain does help the clinician with initial empiric therapy.

Community-Acquired Pneumonia
Lung infection that occurs outside of a hospital or other institution. Common
organisms are as follows:
- *Streptococcus pneumoniae*   - *Hemophilus influenzae*
- *Staphylococcus aureus*   - *Moraxella catarrhalis*

Assess PORT risk classification
The PORT risk classification system is a point scale, with each risk factor adding up
points, as noted above. The classification is as follows:
- Classes I and II   ≤ 70 points
(Class I would be a more obviously well-appearing pt)
- Class III   71–90 points
- Class IV   91–130 points
- Class V   > 130 points

Differential diagnosis
- Nosocomial pneumonia   - Aspiration pneumonia   - Asthma
- Lung cancer   - Tuberculosis   - Pulmonary
- CHF   embolism

P **Treat pts in risk classes I to III with outpatient antibiotic therapy and follow up**
Prescribe a macrolide, doxycycline, or fluoroquinolone.
- Alternatives would include amoxicillin-clavulanate or a 2nd-/3rd-generation oral cephalosporin.
Stress that the antibiotic regimen must be completed, even if the pt feels better early on
in the course of treatment.
Consider treating pts in class III with a brief inpatient observation period if warranted.

Admit pts in risk class IV to the inpatient medical ward, culture, and treat with broad-spectrum antibiotics
Obtain two sets of blood cultures, before treatment with either a fluoroquinolone
alone, or a 2nd-/3rd-generation cephalosporin with a macrolide.
Alternately, consider ampicilin/sulbactam or piperacillin/tazobactam with a macrolide.

Admit pts in risk class V to the intensive care unit, culture, and treat with broad-spectrum antibiotics
Antibiotic choices will include 2nd-/3rd-generation cephalosporin or β-lactam/
β-lactamase inhibitor with a fluoroquinolone or macrolide.

Later, tailor antibiotic treatment based on sputum culture and sensitivities
These will help reduce the emergence of resistant organisms.

Provide high-risk pts with prophylaxis from infections with pneumococcal and influenza vaccines
High-risk pts include those older than age 65, immunocompromised pts, and those
with chronic illnesses mentioned above.

Consider CXR follow-up in 6 wks
This is the minimum time that you would expect to visualize total resolution of a
successfully treated infiltrate. Persistence of infiltrates beyond this time warrants
additional workup of either incomplete treatment or other etiologies.

S   **Does the pt have episodic dyspnea, cough, wheezing, and/or chest tightness?**
These are classic symptoms of asthma and are often worse at night or in the early morning.
Characterized by reversibility of symptoms following bronchodilator therapy.

How often do symptoms occur? Do they occur at night?
This will help classify the severity of chronic asthma (Table 2).

How often is the pt admitted to the ER for asthma? Has the pt been intubated?
This will also give some idea of the severity of the pt's asthma.

Does the pt have exposure to possible triggers of asthma?
- Exercise   - Sinusitis   - GERD
- Cigarette smoke   - Aspiration   - Smog
- Sulfates   - Nitrates   - Allergens
- NSAIDs

O   **Conduct a PE and ABG to classify the severity of the current asthma exacerbation (Table 3)**
Order a chest x-ray
Although you may see only hyperinflation, bronchial wall thickening, and peripheral lung shadows, you may also be able to rule out pneumonia and pneumothorax.

A   **Asthma**
Inflammatory disease of the lung characterized by reversible airway obstruction
Classify the asthma severity as mild intermittent, mild persistent, moderate persistent, or severe persistent.
Also note whether the pt's asthma is stable on this visit or whether the pt is having an exacerbation.

Differential diagnosis
- Foreign body aspiration   - Tracheal stenosis   - Cystic fibrosis
- Chronic bronchitis   - Bronchiolitis obliterans   - Churg-Strauss
- Bronchiectasis   - Allergic bronchopulmonary   syndrome
                              aspergillosis

P   **If the pt is not currently having an asthma exacerbation, or if it is mild, prescribe the appropriate medications based on the severity of the asthma**
Mild Intermittent: Albuterol as needed
Mild Persistent: Add a low-dose inhaled corticosteroid twice daily.
Moderate Persistent: Increase the dose of corticosteroids to medium or add a long-acting β_2 agonist. A leukotriene antagonist or theophylline may substitute for the long-acting β_2 agonist daily.

Table 2 Asthma Classification		
Category	**Symptoms**	**Nighttime Symptoms**
Mild intermittent	$\leq 2 \times$ /week	$\leq 2 \times$ /month
Mild persistent	$> 2 \times$ /week, but $< 1 \times$ /day	$> 2 \times$ /month
Moderate persistent	Daily symptoms	$> 1 \times$ /week
Severe persistent	Continual symptoms	Frequent

Table 3 Asthma Exacerbation				
	Mild	**Moderate**	**Severe**	**Impending Resp. Failure**
Speech	Sentences	Phrases	Words	Mute
Body position	Can be supine	Prefers sitting	Unable to be supine	Unable to be supine
Respiratory rate	Normal	Increased	> 30/min	> 30 min
Breath sounds	Mod. wheezes late expiration	Loud wheezes through expiration	Loud insp. exp. wheezes	Little air movement
Heart rate	< 100 bpm	100–120	> 120	Relatively slow
Mental status	May be agitated	Agitated	Agitated	Drowsy
Peak Expirtory Flow (% predicted)	> 80	50–80	< 50	< 50
SaO_2 (% room air)	> 95	91–95	< 91	< 91
PaO_2 (mm Hg, room air)	Normal	> 60	< 60	< 60
$PaCO_2$ (mm Hg)	< 42	< 42	≥ 42	≥ 42

Severe Persistent: High-dose inhaled corticosteroids and a long-acting β_2 agonist twice daily. Add oral corticosteroids as needed. Attempts should be made to reduce corticosteroid dosages at every visit during which symptoms are well controlled.

Admit pts with evidence of moderate to severe asthma exacerbation to the hospital
Frequent high-dose delivery of inhaled short-acting β_2 agonists, either as metered-dose inhaler or as nebulizer, with at least three doses in the first hr.
Systemic corticosteroids and mucolytics should also be given to these pts.

Intubate those pts with severe asthma with poor or slow response to treatment and start mechanical ventilation
Further management should ensure adequate oxygenation, avoidance of barotrauma, and hypotension.
Administer inhaled short-acting β_2 agonists and systemic anti-inflammatory medications frequently.

Discharge when
Hypoxia and all other signs of respiratory distress are resolved.

Prescribe a dose of oral prednisone tapered from 60 mg po qd over the next 5 days
Consider outpatient pulmonary function testing when asymptomatic to document severity of disease and response to bronchodilator.
This will also help rule out COPD.

S Does the pt have risk factors for contracting tuberculosis (TB)?
- Recent contact with TB - Homelessness - Overcrowded housing
- Incarceration - HIV - Immunosuppressive therapy

Does the pt come from Latin America or Southeast Asia? Does he or she have a history of previous incomplete treatment for TB? Has he or she had exposure to someone with documented drug-resistant TB?

These questions are crucial to ask, because they can point out someone who is at risk of carrying multidrug-resistant tuberculosis (MDRTB).

Does the pt have symptoms consistent with TB?
- Malaise - Anorexia - Weight loss
- Night sweats - Chronic cough - Blood-streaked sputum
- Fevers

Although these symptoms are not specific to tuberculosis, together they suggest the possibility of TB.

Weight loss and night sweats are slightly more specific to TB, but the most common presentation is a chronic cough.

The pt may have no symptoms at all, as in latent tubercular infections.

 Perform PE

Pertinent findings include cachexia, fever, rales, and decreased breath sounds.
- These are nonspecific findings.

Expect that a pt with latent TB might have an entirely normal PE.

Obtain CXR

Primarily important in distinguishing latent TB from reactivation/active TB.

Primary TB shows infiltrate with hilar lymphadenopathy. It rarely presents as a pathologic state. Often the pt is not even aware of it.

Residual (healed)/latent TB would show a primary calcified focus (Ghon focus) with or without calcified hilar lymphadenopathy (Ranke complex).
- Calcified foci are sometimes referred to as granulomata.

Reactivation TB (common active disease) usual presents as infiltrates in the apical posterior segments of the upper lobe or superior segment of lower lobes.

TB can present as multiple nodular densities (military TB), which suggests hematologic and lymphatic dissemination. Other findings include pleural effusion, scarring, and volume loss.

If you suspect active TB, order a sputum sample with a smear for acid-fast bacilli (AFB) and culture for TB. Repeat twice more every 8 hrs for a total of three specimens

Although the culture may not grow out for 6 to 12 wks, the AFB smear, if positive, will confirm the presence of active TB.

Sputum induction may help achieve specimens in pts who cannot provide specimens.
- If induction is not an option, bronchoscopy may also be used to obtain samples.

Place a tuberculin skin test in relevant individuals

This would include pts who have symptoms of TB or asymptomatic people who you are concerned may have latent TB.

Place 5 tuberculin units of protein purified derivative (PPD) on the volar aspect of the forearm, and measure the area of induration (NOT erythema) after 48 to 72 hrs.

Positive tests are interpreted differently for different populations:

- >5 mm: (+) in HIV-positive pts, recent contacts of active TB, signs of previous TB on CXR, and immunosuppressed pts
- >10 mm: (+) in recent immigrants from Asia, Africa, Latin America, HIV-negative injection drug users, TB lab personnel, residents and employees of high-risk settings (e.g., nursing homes, AIDS facilities, homeless shelters, jails), children < 4 years old, or minors exposed to adults at high risk
- > 15 mm: (+) in anyone

A Tuberculosis

The tuberculin bacillus is inhaled and taken to the deepest part of the lungs. In most people, primary infection is rapidly contained by the immune system, but the acid-fast covering of the bacillus renders it difficult to kill by macrophages. This is latent tuberculosis infection.

The bacillus can live inside a macrophage for years, waiting for the moment when the host's immune system is less active. Then reactivation occurs, usually in areas of highest oxygen tension (the upper lobes of the lungs).

Reactivation disease is often more severe than primary, and immune activity causes cavitation in the lungs with caseation necrosis on pathology.

- Note that reactivation can occur in any part of the body, including the peritoneum, pleura, meninges, and kidneys.

Differential diagnosis

- Pneumonia   - Coccidioidomycosis   - Histoplasmosis
- Sarcoidosis   - Blastomycosis   - Lung cancer

P Immediately isolate those you suspect of having active TB

Respiratory isolation is required to prevent spread of infection.
Obtain three samples of sputum for AFB smears.
If they are all negative, you can remove the pt from isolation.

Begin treatment for those with active TB

Common antituberculosis medications include Rifampin (R), Isoniazid/INH (I), Pyrazinamide (P), Ethambutol (E), and Streptomycin (S).
Start R.I.P.E. until culture and sensitivities return.

- If cultures return with INH-sensitive TB, then give R.I.P. for 2 months and then R.I. for an additional 4 months or until follow-up AFB cultures are negative for 3 months, whichever is longer.
- If cultures return with INH-resistant TB, then give R.P. and either E. or S. for 6 months or 12 months of R.E. Remember that streptomycin is given intravenously only.
- If cultures return with MDRTB, a minimum of three drugs (that it is susceptible to) are required with directly observed therapy until culture is negative, and then continue with two drugs for another 12 months.

If pregnant, give R.I.E. for 9 months and do not allow breastfeeding.
Pts with HIV are treated in similar fashion as described but require treatment of longer duration and should be given pyridoxine (Vitamin B_6) to reduce INH-induced peripheral neuropathy.

Begin treatment for those with latent TB (PPD+, CXR negative, or with evidence of old disease)

I. for 9 months OR
R.P. for 2 months if contact of person with known MDRTB

S Does the pt exhibit any suggestive symptoms?

Symptoms can be varied and nonspecific. They include:

- Dyspnea   - Pleuritic chest pain   - Tachypnea
- Fever   - Anxiety

These nonspecific complaints not only make the diagnosis difficult to pinpoint, but they also result in the high level of mortality in these pts. Therefore, keep a high index of suspicion in any pt with risk factors for venous thromboembolism!

Does the pt have any risk factors for deep vein thrombosis (DVT)?

See Deep Vein Thrombosis (p. 98).

O Perform physical exam

- Increased respiratory rate   - Decreased O_2 saturation   - Tachycardia
- Hypotension   - Low-grade fever   (most common)
- Loud pulmonary component of S_2

Obtain an ECG

Classic signs only seen in approximately 5% of pts:

- Right ventricular strain   - Right bundle branch block
- Right axis deviation
- S1Q3T3: S-wave in lead I, Q-wave in lead III, and T-wave inversion in lead III

Very often the only signs will be sinus tachycardia with nonspecific T-wave changes.

Obtain CXR

Prominent pulmonary vasculature (Westermark sign) and increased opacity at the pleural areas second to bleeding (Hamptom hump) are classic signs but are rarely seen.

Most commonly, CXR will be normal.

Perform an arterial blood gas (ABG)

Signs include acute respiratory alkalosis and hypoxia with an increased A-a gradient.

Send serum for D-dimers (the products made by Factor XIII when clot is formed)

If negative, rules out pulmonary embolism (PE) in low-risk pts. A positive study is fairly nonspecific.

Obtain a ventilation-perfusion (V/Q) scan

Radiolabeled albumin is injected into the venous system and is compared with inhaled radioactive gases. Look for defects in perfusion relative to ventilation to generate a high, low, or intermediate probability of a PE.

- Can only be done if CXR is normal.

Normal excludes PE and high probability rules in PE. Low or intermediate probability with high clinical suspicion should lead to an ultrasound or pulmonary angiogram (see below).

A good alternative to the V/Q scan is the computed tomography pulmonary angiogram of the chest. It can be used even if the CXR is abnormal

Uses radio-opaque dye and serial CT images of the chest to define proximal pulmonary vessel thromboembolism. It has low sensitivity for distant, segmental embolisms.

A good adjunctive study is the venous duplex ultrasound of the legs

This is because approximately 70% of cases of PE will have a DVT.

Rarely, a pulmonary angiogram will be necessary
This test is the gold standard that will identify the intraluminal filling defects, arterial abrupt cutoffs, or slow filling that would suggest PE, but it is a much more invasive study.

Pulmonary Embolism
Identify your clinical suspicion as high, intermediate, or low.

Pulmonary embolism occurs when an insoluble mass (usually a thrombus, but this can also include fat, air, tumor, talc, or amniotic fluid) travels through the venous system to the right side of the heart and is carried through to the pulmonary vasculature. It then becomes lodged in the largest vessel that can accommodate it. The following effects result:

- *Increased pulmonary vascular resistance*: caused by obstruction and serotonin secretion.
- *Impaired gas exchange*: multiple reasons, but mainly caused by right-to-left shunting
- *Alveolar hypoventilation*: because the irritant receptors are reflexively stimulated
- *Increased airway resistance*: because bronchoconstriction also occurs
- *Decreased pulmonary compliance*: because lung edema occurs with surfactant loss

All of this leads to right ventricular dysfunction.

If a pulmonary embolus occurs in the most proximal vasculature, death may result.

Differential diagnosis
- Myocardial infarction
- COPD
- CHF
- Anxiety
- Angina
- Asthma
- Pneumothorax
- Pneumonia
- Pericarditis
- Costochondritis

Give pt supplemental oxygen
Preferably through face mask rather than nasal cannula. Intubate if necessary.

If PE likely, begin anticoagulation with heparin, unfractionated
80 units/kg IV bolus then 18 units/kg/hr infusion.
Check PTT in 6 hrs and readjust infusion for goal PTT ratio of 1.5 to 2.5.

Once heparin started, start concurrent warfarin therapy
Adjust daily dose until INR goal ratio of 2.0 to 3.0, at which time heparin infusion may stop.
Continue treatment for 6 months.

Consider low-molecular-weight heparin injections in place of warfarin in pregnancy
Warfarin is a potent teratogen.

Consider thrombolytic therapy with alteplase, streptokinase, or urokinase in pts with documented PEs who are hemodynamically unstable
Contraindications include stroke, active internal bleeding, or surgery or trauma within the past 6 wks.

Monitor pts on heparin for heparin-induced thrombocytopenia and bleeding. Consider inferior vena cava filter placement for pts with contraindications to anticoagulation

S **Is there any progressive dyspnea and nonproductive cough?**
These are the classic symptoms of interstitial lung disease (ILD).

Are there any occupational and environmental exposures?
The potential causes for ILD number more than 100. A good history is crucial to developing a possible etiology. Possible causes include:

- Asbestosis   - Organic gases   - Berylliosis
- Silicosis   - Pneumoconiosis

Is there a history of granulomatous lung diseases?
Sarcoid, fungal, or mycobacterial infections are all associated with ILDs.

What are the pt's past and current medication?
Agents known to cause ILD include:

- Bleomycin   - Busulfan   - Methotrexate
- Chlorambucil   - Cyclophosphamide - Carmustine
- Amiodarone   - Sulfonamides   - Gold salts

Is there any history of connective tissue disorders?
- Lupus   - Rheumatoid arthritis   - Dermatomyositis
- Wegener granulomatosis   - Goodpasture syndrome

Is there any exposure to radiation?
Radiation pneumonitis can also cause ILD.

O **Auscultate the lungs**
Distinctive dry rales ("Velcro sound") are characteristic for ILD.

Observe for evidence of hypoxemia
Low resting pulse oximetry reading, high respiratory rate, cyanosis, or clubbing

Observe any evidence of right-sided heart failure
Elevated neck veins and edema. Often the result of secondary pulmonary hypertension.

Review the CXR
Although x-rays may be normal in some pts, very often there are usually early (ground-glass) or late (coarse reticular pattern) findings of ILD. Additional findings may suggest a certain etiology for ILD:

- *Pleural disease*: asbestosis, radiation pneumonitis, systemic rheumatic disease
- *Hilar/mediastinal lymphadenopathy*: berylliosis, sarcoidosis, silicosis, amyloidosis, lymphocytic interstitial pneumonia
- *Upper lung involvement*: berylliosis, silicosis, ankylosing spondylitis, chronic hypersensitivity pneumonitis

Perform an ABG and pulmonary function test (PFT)
Although an ABG might be normal, hypoxemia is seen later on.

PFT revealing a decreased total lung volume and vital capacity with increased diffusion capacity of the lungs are associated with ILD. This is known as a restrictive pattern on PFT.

Interstitial Lung Disease
There are many forms of ILD, but they all have one thing in common: progressive, diffuse pulmonary scarring. This scarring reduces the lungs' ability to expand and oxygenate normally, thus producing the restrictive pattern noted above.

The most common form of ILD is idiopathic pulmonary fibrosis, which occurs usually in the sixth decade of life but can occur in any age group. It is an immune-mediated disease in which injury occurs to the type I alveolar cells, and fibroblast growth and production is stimulated, thus leading to scarring.

Other forms of ILD include
All of the exposures noted above, lupus, rheumatoid arthritis, ankylosing spondylitis, Goodpasture syndrome, sarcoidosis, pulmonary alveolar proteinosis, eosinophilic pneumonias, and lymphangiomyomatosis

Differential diagnosis
Always consider tuberculosis, *Pneumocystis carinii* pneumonia, and lymphangitic metastases of malignancy.

P **Perform workup to discover cause of ILD**
A thorough workup of ILD should include:
- C-ANCA to help rule out Wegener granulomatosis
- An antiglomerular basement membrane to rule out Goodpasture syndrome
- Bronchoscopy with bronchoalveolar lavage to look for lymphocytic or neutrophilic dominant cells in the lavage
- CT scan of chest, and consider using high resolution
- Biopsy (open lung or transbronchial) to rule out carcinoma and identify the etiologic agent if diagnosis remains in doubt

Begin by treating both the underlying pathophysiology and providing symptomatic relief
Treat/remove underlying agent.

Provide supplemental oxygen to correct hypoxemia. Make arrangements for home O_2 if severe enough.

If an autoimmune cause is suspected, corticosteroids will likely be necessary
Prednisone at 1 mg/kg daily for 8 wks followed by a maintenance dose of 0.25 mg/kg/day for at least 6 months

If the disease persists, consider cyclophosphamide
Start at 1 mg/kg/day while continuing the prednisone.

Cyclophosphamide doses can be increased by approximately 50 mg/day titrating to a WBC count approximately half of normal baseline in an attempt to suppress lymphocyte activity. Hold for neutrophil counts < 1000.

Make arrangements for lung transplantation in pts with progressive or end-stage ILD

S   **Does the pt smoke cigarettes? If so, for how many years and how many packs smoked per day?**

Approximately 25% of all solitary pulmonary nodules noted on chest x-ray (CXR) are found to be malignant. An accurate smoking history may indicate a level of suspicion of primary lung cancer.

Ask if the pt has any other history of cancer

This nodule may also represent a nonlung malignancy that has metastasized to the lungs, such as colon, breast, cervix, prostate, ovary, stomach, or bladder cancer. Usually, however, these will present with multiple bilateral nodules.

Ask if the pt has any history of tuberculosis, coccidiomycoses, histoplasmosis, or sarcoidoisis

A significant portion of "benign" lung nodules (~75%) can be linked to fungal or mycobacterial infections or granulomatous reactions.
Other benign nodules include hamartomas.

Has the pt had any fevers, night sweats, or weight loss?

These are the common "B" symptoms and are associated with both malignancy and with granulomatous diseases such as tuberculosis.

What is the pt's age?

In general, malignancies are less likely in pts who are younger than 35 years old.

O   **PE will usually reveal nonspecific findings. Nevertheless, note the following**

Pt's temperature, other vital signs, and overall appearance (cachetic?)
Check for palpable lymphadenopathy.
Observation of respirations, palpation, percussion, and auscultation of lungs
For men, digital rectal exam; for women, breast exam and cervical exam with PAP smear

Obtain CXR

A current chest radiograph compared to an older film (ideally 2 years ago) can provide important clues regarding the possibility of malignancy.

Size:
- 2–5 mm → 1% chance of malignancy
- 11–20 mm → 33% chance of malignancy
- 21–45 mm → 80% chance of malignancy

Estimation of doubling time:
- < 30 days suggests infection
- > 2 years suggests benign hamartoma or granuloma

Nodule edge:
- Smooth and well-defined suggests benign etiology.
- Ill-defined and lobular suggests malignancy.

High-resolution computed tomography of the chest can provide additional clues of etiology and guide management

Calcifications:
- Central and lamellar calcifications suggests benign etiology.
- Sparse and eccentric calcifications suggests malignancy.

Appearance:
- Spiculated, peripheral halos, or thick wall cavitary lesion also suggest malignancy.

Location:
- Peripheral lesions are easier to biopsy with transthoracic needle aspiration.
- Central lesions, especially with mediastinal lymphadenopathy, can be biopsied by bronchoscopy or thoracoscopy.

Consider performing a PET scan if available
Operates by sensing glucose metabolism of cells
Prized for its high sensitivity and specificity in detecting malignancy
Poor sensitivity if lesion is small (< 1 cm)
Expensive

Solitary Pulmonary Nodule
Although this general diagnosis is sufficient while a workup is in progress, it is a good idea to comment on the likelihood (low, medium, or high) of malignancy.
- A pt younger than 30 years of age, with a stable lung nodule over 2 years with a central calcification pattern would be considered a <u>low</u> probability of malignancy.
- A 60-year-old, 40 pack-year smoker with a new lung nodule in the last year, 5 cm in size, with a lobular pattern on CXR and sparse, eccentric calcification pattern would be considered a <u>high</u> probability of malignancy.

Pts with a <u>low</u> probability of malignancy can be followed with serial CXRs every 3 months for the first year and then every 6 months for the second year
This follow-up should be sufficient to establish the benignity of the lesion.

Pts with a <u>high</u> probability of malignancy can proceed directly to surgical resection without biopsy, so long as it is not contraindicated
Pulmonary function tests will have to be performed to establish that the pt can tolerate lung surgery.
This will allow for biopsy and resection at the same time.

The remaining pts with <u>intermediate</u> probability will have to undergo biopsy for definitive diagnosis. Each method has its own benefits and risks
Transthoracic needle aspiration, CT-guided
- Higher diagnostic yield then bronchoscopy for peripherally located masses
- Higher complication rate, such as pneumothorax
- Higher false-negative rate, operator-dependent associated error

Bronchoscopy
- Better suited for centrally located lesions, particularly with lymphadenopathy

III

Cardiology

S   Have the pt describe the pain and where it is located

Rule out life-threatening causes first before considering more benign conditions.

Myocardial infarction (MI) or unstable angina present with pain referred over precordium with occasional referral to left arm, jaw, and chin.

- *Unstable angina*: Characterized by chest discomfort that is provoked by less exertion than before. Usually relieved by rest and or nitroglycerin (NTG).
- *MI*: characterized by chest pain lasting > 30 min that is not relieved by NTG.

Stable angina presents with similar discomfort, but is consistently provoked by the same level of exertion, lasts only 3 to 10 min, and is relieved with rest and NTG.

Gastroesophageal reflux is usually accompanied by a sour taste in the mouth, worse with reclining or supine position after meals.

Pulmonary embolism (PE), pneumothorax (PTX), aortic dissection, pneumonia, and pericarditis can all present with sharp pain on inspiration (pleuritic).

- *Pulmonary embolism, pneumothorax*: sudden onset with dyspnea
- *Aortic dissection*: sudden onset with tearing sensation to the back between the scapulae
- *Pneumonia*: more gradual in onset with rigors and cough with purulent sputum

What potential risk factors does the pt have for these diseases?

Cardiac diseases:

- Hypertension	- Diabetes	- Hyperlipidemia
- Cigarette use	- Cocaine use	- History of arrhythmias
- Atrial fibrillation	- Aortic stenosis	- Other valvular
- Past MI	- Coronary artery disease	abnormalities

Pulmonary embolus:

| - Prolonged immobilization or rest | - Oral contraceptive use |
| - History of neoplasm/cancer | - Recent trauma or surgery |

Pneumothorax:

| - COPD | - Marfan syndrome |
| - Cigarette use | - Asthma |

The only known risk for aortic dissection is uncontrolled hypertension.

O   Perform a physical exam focused on potential cardiac and pulmonary causes

Vital signs:

- Rapid heart rate and low blood pressure: acute coronary syndrome, PTX, or PE.
- Hypertension is nonspecific but indicates a potential cardiac cause.
- Tachypnea/poor O_2 sats indicate pulmonary causes such as PE, PTX, or pneumonia, but can also be a sign of cardiogenic shock causing pulmonary congestion and edema.

Neck:

- Holosystolic murmur in the carotids: aortic stenosis
- Elevated neck veins: right heart congestion indicating an acute coronary event, valvular abnormality, pericardial tamponade, pulmonary embolism, or pneumothorax

Chest:

- Decreased/absent breath sounds: PTX; confirm with hyperresonance to percussion.

- Rales: left ventricular failure
- Sharp pain to palpation: costochondritis, broken rib (palpation reproduces pain), or herpes zoster (may see vesicles and erythema in a dermatomal pattern)

Heart:

- Displaced apex with sustained heave: left ventricular hypertrophy
- Loud pulmonary component of S_2: pulmonary embolism
- S_3: volume overload
- S_4: pressure overload
- Friction rubs: pericarditis
- Systolic murmur: aortic stenosis, mitral regurgiation, or tachycardia
- Diastolic murmur: mitral stenosis or aortic regurgitation

Ext:

- Peripheral edema: right ventricular failure
- Asymmetric pulses: aortic dissection

A Chest pain

Not all that causes chest pain is cardiac in origin. Consider all of the following sites:

- Skin	- Chest/back muscles	- Ribs/costochondral joints
- Pleura	- Pericardium	- Esophagus
- Aorta	- Ischemic myocardium	

- Referred pain from stomach, gallbladder, or pancreas

P Order a CXR and stat ECG

ECG:

- ST-segment depression: ischemia
- ST-segment elevation: infarction, or if diffuse, pericarditis
- Right axis deviation, right bundle branch block, and right ventricular hypertrophy: pulmonary embolism

CXR:

- Collapsed lung field/Hyperlucency: pneumothorax
- Engorged central pulmonary vasculature: pulmonary embolus
- Widened mediastinum: aortic dissection
- Cardiomegaly: left ventricular hypertrophy, congestive heart failure (CHF), and valvular disorders
- Pulmonary edema: CHF
- Infiltrates: pneumonia
- Rib fractures should be apparent.

Begin immediate empiric treatment based on working diagnosis

Stable angina: give nitroglycerin, β-blocker, aspirin. Order troponin q4h × 3.

Acute coronary syndrome: nitroglycerin, oxygen, morphine, aspirin, β-blocker, and heparin. Order troponin q4h × 3. If ST-elevation MI, consider pt's eligibility for cardiac catheterization. (See Acute Coronary Syndromes, p. 34.)

Pulmonary embolism: O_2, heparin, then warfarin; thrombolytics if unstable

Pneumothorax: oxygen followed by chest tube placement

- *Tension PTX*: Place needle in chest on affected side at midaxillary line of 4th intercostal space.

Aortic dissection: β-blocker, morphine, stat CT chest with IV contrast to confirm diagnosis. Call cardiothoracic surgery.

Costochondritis: NSAID therapy only.

S **Is the pt's pain quality and duration characteristic of stable angina?**
The pain classically should be dull tightness, squeezing, or pressure sensation over the
precordium or left side of chest with occasional radiation to left arm, jaw, or chin.
It should last 3 to 10 minutes and be relieved by rest.
If it lasts greater than 30 minutes, consider an acute coronary syndrome (ACS).

Is the pain precipitated consistently with the same amount of exertion?

Pts with stable angina present with symptoms that are evoked by the same level of
activity (e.g., climbing two flights of stairs or walking more than 60 feet at a time).
The consistency is very important.

If the pt provides a history of requiring less activity now to evoke the same symptoms,
the pt is experiencing unstable angina, which is treated very differently.

What makes the discomfort better?
Stable angina is usually relieved by rest or with sublingual nitroglycerin.
• These are classic symptoms, and deviation from this pattern is important.
• Pts with symptoms of stable angina that fail to be relieved with three doses of
  nitroglycerin need to be evaluated for an ACS.

Does the pt have any cardiac risk factors?
- Diabetes mellitus   - Hypertension   - Hyperlipidemia
- Post-myocardial infarction - Cigarette use   - Cocaine use

O **Perform a PE**
Although the PE may be normal in an asymptomatic pt, you might see hypo-/
hypertension, tachycardia, or systolic murmurs or gallops during an ischemic episode.
The PE is also useful for revealing any other evidence of disease that could contribute to
coronary artery disease, such as diabetes mellitus (neuropathy, retinopathy), thyroid
disease, or hypertension.

Obtain an ECG
Although the ECG can be normal in asymptomatic pts, the classic findings are
ST-segment depression of at least 1 mm that is downward sloping during the ischemic
episode and resolves after symptoms disappear.
Findings may be nonspecific, such as T-wave flattening or inversion.
ST-elevations indicate a myocardial infarction (MI), and this needs to be addressed
very differently and immediately.

**Consider a stress ECG, echocardiography, or scintigraphic imaging
of the heart**
These studies may be performed on an outpatient basis to evaluate for level of activity
tolerance, ejection fraction, wall motion abnormalities, valvular dysfunction, or
territories of affected vessels.

Remember not to let any pt with a history of aortic stenosis perform a stress test.
Sudden death may occur.

A **Stable Angina**

Stable angina occurs when there is a fixed narrowing of a coronary vessel. When at rest, the myocardium is able to obtain all of the blood, and thus oxygen, that it needs through this stenotic region. However, at increased rates of activity and metabolic demand, not enough oxygen reaches the myocardium through this lesion, and symptoms of ischemia (angina) occur.

Again, be sure to distinguish this diagnosis from ACS, which includes unstable angina or ST-elevation MI, which warrants prompt medical attention.

P **Treat acute symptoms with sublingual nitroglycerin**

Administer sublingual nitroglycerin every 3 to 5 minutes until symptoms resolve for up to three doses. If there is no relief, begin a workup and treatment to rule out ACS.

If asymptomatic, give pharmacologic treatment to prevent further episodes of angina

β-blockers: These are first-line agents for treating ischemia because they reduce myocardial oxygen demand by reducing heart rate and afterload.
  • Avoid in pts with reactive airway disease, bradycardia, or congestive heart failure (CHF) exacerbation.

Long-acting nitrates: Isosorbide mononitrate or dinitrate are examples.
  • These doses can be increased and adjusted to reduce symptoms.
  • Be sure to watch for hypotension, headaches, and tolerance to nitrates in these pts.
  • Nitrates have no effects on mortality in this disease, only on the symptoms.

Sublingual nitroglycerin: Either as a spray or tablet, this medicine can be useful for any "breakthrough" symptoms that may occur during an acute attack or as prophylaxis before strenuous activity.
  • A three-dose limit still applies.

Aspirin: This will exhibit antiplatelet activity but should be avoided in those with aspirin-sensitive allergies.
  • In those cases, ticlopidine or clopidogrel may be considered.

Calcium channel blockers: These are reserved more as third-line agents, particularly because of their negative effects in pts with a history of CHF or MI.
  • They are the first-line therapy in pts with Prinzmetal's angina or coronary vasospasm. This phenomenon occurs when the pt has no stenotic coronary lesion but intermittently has angina, usually at rest, caused by coronary spasm.

Modify cardiac risk factors

This means that conditions such as hyperlipidemia, diabetes mellitus, hypertension, smoking, cocaine use, and hyperthyroidism should be medically optimized.

Fasting lipids, glucose, HgbA1C, TSH may be useful lab studies to order from time to time on your pts.

Consider revascularization for pts who still have symptoms despite maximum medical therapy, in post-MI or unstable angina pts with evidence of ischemia despite symptom control

Revascularization would include the evaluation of coronary artery bypass grafting or percutaneous transluminal, coronary angiography with or without stenting.

S **Ask the pt to describe the chest pain**

Acute coronary syndrome (ACS) pain is usually substernal chest pain/discomfort lasting longer than 15 minutes with little relief from nitroglycerin.

Sharp or stabbing pain lasting seconds located to the extreme sides of the chest (right or left) is less likely to be associated with an ACS.

Does the pain radiate to any other part of the body?

In ACS the pain often radiates down the left arm and shoulder, neck, and jaw.

Does the pt have any other symptoms associated with the pain?

- Nausea/vomiting   - Diaphoresis   - Palpitations
- Dizziness   - Shortness of breath

Has the pt ever smoked?

Smoking is one of the top risk factors for ACS.

Does the pt have a history of any other medical problems?

- Hypertension   - Diabetes mellitus   - Hyperlipidemia

Does the pt have any family history of heart disease?

A history of coronary artery disease in a first-degree relative is a significant risk factor for ACS, especially if the family member had his or her first coronary event at a young age ($<$ 50 y/o).

O **Determine the age and sex of the pt**

Males $>$ 55 years or females $>$ 65 years are at increased risk of ACS.

Perform a focused PE, looking for the following symptoms consistent with ACS

Vital signs: tachycardia, hypertension, hypotension

Gen: diaphoresis, anxiety, pallor

Heart: distant heart sounds, murmur, S_3, displaced point of maximal impulse

Lung: rales

Ext: edema, weak distal pulses

Obtain a stat ECG

ST-segment depression indicates ischemia.

ST-segment elevation indicates ongoing infarction (myocardial death).

- The leads displaying ST-segment elevation suggest the affected cardiac walls and, thereby, the affected arteries.
  - V1, V2, V3, V4: septal
  - V5, V6: lateral
  - II, III, avF: inferior

Send serum for stat cardiac enzymes

Troponin I and creatine kinase MB (CK-MB) are released into circulation when cardiac tissue is damaged.

Detection of these enzymes confirms myocardial damage.

- Check troponin I every 4 to 6 hrs times three.
- May check CK-MB every 4 to 8 hrs times three.

Obtain a stat chest radiograph

Cardiomegaly suggests long-standing hypertension or mitral valve dysfunction.

Pulmonary edema suggests left ventricular dysfunction.

Acute Coronary Syndromes

When a section of myocardium is not receiving sufficient blood supply, and therefore oxygen, symptoms of angina (chest pressure, shortness of breath) will result.

Classification of ACSs
Unstable angina:
- Coronary plaque rupture ≡ rapidly stenosing vessel
- Symptoms with decreasing amount of exercise

Non-ST-elevation myocardial infarction (MI):
- Elevated troponin I or CK-MB
- No ST-segment elevation on ECG

ST-elevation MI:
- ST-segment elevations
- Elevated troponin I or CK-MB fraction

Differential diagnosis
Pulm: asthma, COPD; pneumonia, pleurisy, pneumothorax, pulmonary embolism
Cardiac: pericarditis, aortic dissection, stable angina
GI: esophageal spasm, GERD; peptic ulcer disease
Musculoskeletal: costochondritis
Psych: anxiety/panic attack

P **All pts with suspected ACS should be placed on a monitor and begin immediate medical therapy with**

- O_2	- IV fluids	- Aspirin
- Ticlopidine	- Heparin	- Nitroglycerin
- β-blocker	- Morphine	

For ST-elevation MIs, arrange for immediate cardiac catheterization
This will allow a cardiologist to visualize any obstruction in an affected artery and then open the obstruction with balloon angioplasty and a stent.

If catheterization cannot be performed immediately, initiate thrombolytic therapy with streptokinase or tissue plasminogen activator. These clot-dissolving enzymes should effectively open blocked arteries.

With non-ST-elevation MIs or unstable angina, treat medically (see first statement above)

S **Does the pt have symptoms of congestive heart failure (CHF)?**
- Fatigue
- Lethargy
- Dyspnea on exertion
- Paroxysmal nocturnal dyspnea
- Edema

What amount of exertion induces these symptoms?
With greater than normal activity, with normal activity, with minimal activity, or at rest

If the pt has been stable, has there been a rapid deterioration in condition?
Rapid deterioration in an otherwise stable pt with CHF, think of ischemia or infarction of the myocardium.
Gradual deterioration might occur with noncompliance with medication and diet.

Is there any history of hypertension, dilated or restrictive cardiomyopathy, aortic stenosis, hypertrophic cardiomyopathy, myocarditis, or left-sided infarction?
These are common causes of left-sided heart failure.

Is there any history of mitral stenosis, pulmonary hypertension, endocarditis of tricuspid or pulmonary valve, or right ventricular infarction?
These are common causes of right-sided heart failure.

The most common cause of right-sided heart failure is left-sided heart failure.

O **Review vital signs**
Hypertension is a cause of CHF and is common on presentation.
Tachycardia is a compensatory mechanism for volume overload and hypotension.
Tachypnea can be seen with left-sided heart failure as a result of pulmonary edema.

Look for signs of left-sided heart failure
S_3 gallop, rales, wheezes, and murmurs suggestive of mitral and aortic valves

Look for signs of right-sided heart failure
These include elevated jugular venous pressure, lower extremity edema, abnormal hepatojugular reflux, hepatomegaly, and murmurs indicating right-sided heart valves.

Review ECG for signs of CHF
Left ventricular hypertrophy, Q-waves (indicating old transmural infarction), poor R-wave progression (poor LV function), and right ventricular hypertrophy.

Obtain an echocardiogram
Systolic ejection fraction < 40% constitutes moderately reduced systolic function.
Can also reveal wall motion abnormalities, show valvular disorders, show atrial and ventricular size, and reveal right ventricular and pulmonary artery pressures.

A **Congestive Heart Failure**
Inability of the heart to provide enough pressure to move blood. The decreased pressure leads to edema, fluid congestion, and decreased perfusion/oxygen of vital organs.
Most causes include chronic elevated afterload causing weakening of the myocardium.
Symptoms depend on which side of the heart is failing, resulting in either the lungs (left side) or the systemic venous system (right side) being congested with blood.
If possible, further classify whether this represents systolic versus diastolic dysfunction.
Note whether the pt is stable or in CHF exacerbation.

NYHA Classification
Class I: Symptoms only with greater than normal activity
Class II: Symptoms with normal activity
Class III: Symptoms with minimal activity
Class IV: Symptoms at rest

Differential diagnosis
- Acute coronary syndrome   - Pulmonary embolism   - Pneumothorax
- Interstitial lung disease   - Asthma   - Stable angina

Reduce excess intravascular volume
Thiazide diuretics or oral furosemide are suitable for pts with stable CHF.
- Consider IV furosemide if pt is in CHF exacerbation.

Avoid diuretics in pts with diastolic dysfunction because these pts have reduced heart relaxation rather than volume overload. Overdiuresis will lead quickly to hypotension.

Reduce afterload
ACE inhibitors are useful in reducing both afterload and the sympathetic nervous system related to cardiac remodeling. When giving an ACE inhibitor, remember to monitor:
- *Renal function*: Do not to give ACE inhibitors to pts with serum creatinine greater than 2.0.
- *Electrolytes*: Hyperkalemia may occur secondary to aldosterone suppression.

Reduce preload
Pts with CHF will benefit from oral long-acting nitrates. Nitroglycerin as needed is unlikely to help.

In pts with CHF exacerbation, consider IV nitroglycerin; for those with exacerbation and hypertension, sodium nitroprusside has shown to be effective.

Increase cardiac contractility
Digoxin has been used in pts with moderate to severe CHF. Although digoxin has not been shown to actually be of benefit in reducing mortality, it has been shown to improve symptoms and cause fewer admissions related to CHF exacerbation.

Pts with severe CHF admitted to the Cardiac Care Unit with severe hypotension can be treated with IV dobutamine. Use judiciously because oxygen demand can increase with these pts.

Ensure proper oxygenation
As CHF is treated and fluid is removed from the lungs, oxygenation will improve. Until that time, supplemental O_2 should be given to maintain saturation $\geq 95\%$.

When stable, consider addition of low-dose β-blocker (carvedilol) and increase as tolerated

Outpatient therapy should consist of furosemide, ACE inhibitors, and a < 2g/day sodium-restricted diet

S **Does the pt have any risk factors for aortic stenosis (AS)?**
Congenital bicuspid valve or known calcification of aortic valve

Does the pt have any risk factors for mitral valve regurgitation?
Ischemic heart disease:
- Papillary muscle dysfunction
- Ruptured chordae tendineae
- Left ventricular dilation

History of rheumatic fever suggests valvulitis.
Intravenous drug abuse is a risk factor for infective endocarditis.
Illicit diet drugs such as fenfluramine and dexfenfluramine have also been implicated.

Does the pt have angina, syncope, or congestive heart failure?
If the workup reveals aortic stenosis, the average life expectancy is 5 years, 3 years, and 2 years, respectively, without intervention.

Are there other medical problems that increase the risk of a systolic murmur?
Systolic flow murmurs, more common over the aortic or pulmonic valve regions can occur in any hyperdynamic, high-output state (e.g., anemia and hyperthyroidism).

O **Perform a careful exam of the heart. Note where the murmur is best appreciated**
Right upper sternal border: aortic valve   Left upper sternal border: pulmonic valve
Left lower sternal border: tricuspid valve   Apex: mitral valve

Note if the murmur increases with inspiration
This would indicate a right-sided heart murmur (tricuspid or pulmonic).

Note if the murmur is crescendo-decrescendo or holosystolic
Crescendo-decrescendo is the sound of blood being forced across a stenotic opening, thus implicating the pulmonic and aortic valves.
Holosystolic murmurs indicate that blood is regurgitating without resistance, thus implicating the mitral and tricuspid valves and also ventricular septal defects.

Note any preceding midsystolic click or pop
This is a sign of mitral valve prolapse, a myxomatous degeneration of the mitral valve.
The valve is competent at the beginning of systole, but the central portion of the leaflet pops upward into the atrium in midsystole.
If there is no regurgitation, there will only be the click without the murmur.

Have the pt perform the Valsalva maneuver and note if the murmur changes
Murmurs of AS decrease with this maneuver and increase once it is released.
- Valsalva decreases blood flow into the heart (by increasing intrathoracic pressures), thus decreasing the volume of blood crossing the stenotic valve.

Note any change with squatting
AS and mitral regurgitation murmurs both increase with this maneuver, whereas IHSS (a type of cardiomyopathy) will decrease.

Continue listening to the pt's heart as he or she goes from squatting to standing
IHSS murmurs will actually increase, whereas AS murmurs will decrease.

Continue auscultation while pt performs an isometric handgrip
Mitral regurgitation increases with handgrip, whereas AS and IHSS decrease.

Continue auscultation through the respiratory cycle
Tricuspid regurgitation (TR) murmurs should increase with inspiration. Murmurs of pulmonic stenosis and TR should decrease with expiration.

Note if the murmur radiates anywhere
AS should radiate to the carotid arteries.
Mitral regurgitation murmurs often radiate to the axillae.

Note any changes with passive straight-leg raise
AS and TR murmurs tend to increase, whereas IHSS actually decreases.

Palpate the carotid or any other central pulse
AS may have a slow and sustained central pulse (parvus e tardus).

 Systolic murmur
Characterize the murmur as either holosystolic or crescendo-decrescendo.

Differential diagnosis
- Aortic stenosis
- Idiopathic hypertrophic subaortic stenosis
- Tricuspid regurgitation
- Hypertrophic cardiomyopathy
- Benign flow murmur
- Mitral regurgitation
- Pulmonic stenosis
- Ventricular septal defect
- Mitral valve prolapse

P **If you suspect anything other than a flow murmur, order an echocardiogram of the heart**
This study should definitively discern the etiology of the murmur.

For pts with aortic stenosis
Send the pt for cardiac catheterization to measure the pressure gradient across the valve.
- Consider valve replacement if gradient is > 50 mm Hg or valve area is < 1cm.
- Medically manage with diuretics and sodium restriction.
- Digoxin and calcium channel blockers may be used if atrial fibrillation is present.
Advise pt against vigorous aerobic exercise because sudden death may occur.

For pts with mitral regurgitation
Medical management includes diuretics and afterload reduction.
Digoxin and calcium channel blockers may be used for atrial fibrillation.
Schedule mitral valve replacement before irreversible left ventricular dysfunction occurs.

For pulmonic stenosis and tricuspid regurgitation
Intervention is less urgent because right-sided lesions cause less disease.
Refer for replacement when right-sided heart failure symptoms are significant.

For ventricular septal defects
If pulmonary artery pressures are normal on echo, refer these pts for surgery.

For all pts with pathologic murmurs, prescribe antibiotic prophylaxis for dental procedures

S

Does the pt have any risk factors for aortic regurgitation (AR)?
- History of intravenous drug abuse ≡ infective endocarditis
- Congenital bicuspid valve   - Syphilis
- Lupus   - Marfan syndrome

Recent blunt chest trauma (e.g., a steering wheel in a motor vehicle accident) can also be a cause of acute AR.

Does the pt have any risk factors for mitral stenosis (MS)?
Rheumatic fever is the most common cause. Lupus and left atrial myxoma are much more rare.

O

Listen to the heart murmur. Note where it is best appreciated
Right upper sternal border: aortic valve
Left upper sternal border: pulmonic valve
Left lower sternal border: tricuspid valve
Left midaxillary line: mitral valve

Note if the murmur increases with inspiration
This would indicate a right-sided heart murmur.

Note if the murmur is high- or low-pitched
High-pitched murmurs tend to implicate pulmonic and aortic valves, whereas low-pitched murmurs suggest the mitral valve.

Note change with squatting. AR murmur should increase
This is because squatting increases systemic vascular resistance, thus increasing the drive for blood to regurgitate across the aortic valve.

Note change with isometric handgrip
Both AR and MS murmurs should increase.

Note change with breathing
Tricuspid stenosis (TS) murmurs may increase with inspiration and decrease with expiration.

Note change with passive, straight-leg raise
TS murmurs should increase. This is because leg raise increases blood return to the heart, thus causing increased blood flow across the stenotic tricuspid valve.

Look for evidence of mitral stenosis
- Prominent jugular A-waves   - Opening snap
- Diastolic rumble   - Low-pitched
- At apex in left lateral position   - Palpable right ventricular heave
- If severe enough, there may also be evidence of right ventricular dysfunction with bilateral lower extremity edema and ascites.

Look for evidence of aortic regurgitation
Bounding pulses: "water hammer" or Corrigan's pulse
Capillary pulsations of nailbeds with lightly applied pressure (Quincke's sign)
"Bobbing head" in systole (de Musset's sign)
Widened pulse pressure (large difference between systole and diastole)
S_3 on apex
Point of maximal impulse deviated to left and down

Review CXR
Cardiomegaly from left ventricular hypertrophy might be seen with chronic AR. Pulmonary congestion and edema would be seen with chronic MS.

Diastolic murmur
If enough clinical evidence exists, make a working diagnosis on what you believe is the likely etiology.

Differential diagnosis
Aortic regurgitation
Mitral stenosis
Tricuspid stenosis
Pulmonic regurgitation
Atrial septal defect (ASD)

- A congenital ASD can go unnoticed for a lifetime because its characteristic sound, a fixed split S_2, can be difficult to hear, and because as a low-pressure system, it takes a long time for the left-to-right shunt to manifest physical symptoms. However, when enough blood has been shunted to the pulmonary system, the tricuspid valve may experience a relative stenosis. This diastolic murmur may be the first sign of an ASD and may occur relatively late in life.

Order an echocardiogram of the heart
This study should definitively answer the etiology of the murmur.

If the echo reveals aortic regurgitation, begin with medical therapy
Treat congestive heart failure (CHF) symptoms, if present, with ACE inhibitors, diuretics, and sodium restriction.

If medical therapy fails, or if the pt has acute AR with left ventricular failure, either systolic or diastolic, call a cardiothoracic surgery consult
Surgical replacement of the valve will be necessary.

If the echo reveals MS, again begin with medical therapy
Treat atrial fibrillation with rate control and anticoagulation. If CHF is present (almost certainly would be right-sided), treat with diuretics and sodium reduction.

Call a cardiothoracic surgery consult if mitral valve area is < 0.7 cm² or if symptoms persist on maximal medical therapy
It is possible that the stenosis can be relieved without valve replacement, but surgical widening will be necessary. If that fails, the valve will need to be replaced.

Prescribe antibiotic prophylaxis for these pts for all dental procedures
All pts with valvular lesions severe enough to cause a murmur (produced by turbulent blood flow) are at risk for endocarditis.

S **Is the pt experiencing an irregular heart rhythm or palpitations?**
These are the most common symptoms reported by pts.
Asymptomatic atrial fibrillation is even more common.
If the duration is longer than 48 hrs or unknown, evaluate for possible atrial thrombus.

Are there symptoms of shortness of breath, chest pain, or altered mental status?
These symptoms may indicate shock, myocardial infarction, or pulmonary edema.
If they are present, strongly consider urgent cardioversion.

Does the pt have a history of hypertension, coronary artery disease, valvular heart disease, atrial septal defect, hyperthyroidism, pericarditis, or chest surgery?
These are common medical and surgical causes of atrial fibrillation.

Is the pt taking any medications? Does he or she use any drugs or alcohol?
Theophylline and β-agonists are common medications that can cause atrial fibrillation.
Excessive alcohol intake ("holiday heart") is a common cause of atrial fibrillation that is often transient and self-resolving.

Does the pt have a history of congestive heart failure, diabetes, hypertension, valvular disorders, or prior stroke? Is he or she older than 75 years of age?
A "yes" answer to any one of these questions identifies someone who is at significantly increased risk of stroke and should be considered for anticoagulation.

O **Perform a focused PE**

Pulse: A resting heart rate higher than 100 beats per minute is defined as rapid ventricular rate and warrants rate control with medications or cardioversion.

- Note that not all ventricular beats translate into a palpable radial pulse. The difference between the ventricular and radial pulse is known as the "pulse deficit."

Blood pressure: Without atrial systole and with a rapid ventricular rate, stroke volume can fall dramatically. Severe hypotension is an indication for urgent cardioversion.
Lungs: Pulmonary edema, characterized by rales and bibasilar decreased breath sounds, may be another indication for urgent cardioversion.
Heart: The classic finding is an irregularly irregular heart beat.

- An S4 representing an "atrial kick" is, by definition, absent in these pts.

Examine the ECG
Atrial activity should be disorganized, with an atrial rate between 400 to 600 beats per minute. This is represented by the "fibrillating baseline." There will be no discernible P-waves, and their presence should lead you to another diagnosis.
The ventricular rate, represented by QRS complexes, should be irregular. It may or may not be rapid (> 100 bpm).
If the pt has paroxysmal atrial fibrillation, the ECG may be normal.
Evidence of ischemia or infarction on ECG warrants prompt preparation for urgent cardioversion (see Acute Coronary Syndromes, p. 34).

Review the CXR
Evidence of pulmonary congestion or edema warrants urgent cardioversion.

Atrial fibrillation with or without rapid ventricular response
A normally functioning heart should beat approximately 60 to 100 times per minute.
In atrial fibrillation, foci discharge all over the atria and prevent coordinated atrial
contraction.
In general, an adult atrioventricular node will not transmit faster than 160 to 170 beats
per minute, which is why the rate in atrial fibrillation is usually about 160 to 170.

Differential diagnosis
Atrial flutter: very similar to atrial fibrillation and treated the same
  • Characterized by "sawtooth" pattern on ECG
Paroxysmal supraventricular tachycardia: A rapid rate requiring a reentry pathway
around the atrioventricular node. Although there are no P-waves, it should be regular.
Sinus or junctional tachycardias: Monofocal rapid rhythms. P-waves will be present.
Sinus rhythms with premature beats: Premature atrial or ventricular beats; if frequent
enough can make a rhythm seem irregular.

 **If the pt is hemodynamically unstable or has pulmonary edema, he or
she should be admitted and urgently cardioverted, first electrically and
then chemically if unsuccessful**
Electrical cardioversion includes an initial synchronized shock at 100 or 200 Joules
followed by another shock at 360 Joules if unsuccessful.
Chemical cardioversion involves loading and infusion of either ibutilide or
procainamide.

If the pt is stable and has a rapid ventricular response, use medications to control the rate
β-blockers, calcium channel blockers with chronotropic properties (e.g., diltiazem and
verapamil), and digoxin are common rate-control agents used.
  • β-blockers are best suited for those pts with ischemia or infarction.
  • Diltiazem and verapamil will be better suited for those pts with hypertension or
    with contraindications for β-blockers.
These two classes are preferred as initial agents because they can be started
intravenously and switched to oral agents. The following medications should be
considered adjunctive therapy:
  • Digoxin has a slow onset, even with loading.
  • Amiodarone is useful as an adjunct, but again has a slow onset.
Two or three agents may be required to achieve a goal rate of 50 to 100 bpm at rest.

Anticoagulate those pts at risk for thromboembolism
Pts with "lone atrial fibrillation" (< 60 years old and without any risk factors for
stroke) can be managed without anticoagulation or with aspirin alone.
Other pts should be anticoagulated for a minimum period of 3 wks with warfarin with
an international normalized ratio goal of 2.0 to 3.0 before elective cardioversion and
continued for at least 1 month after successful cardioversion.
Otherwise, anticoagulation should be chronic because of increased risk of stroke from
thromboembolism.

Ask the pt to describe the chest pain

The classic characteristics are a sharp chest pain that is worse with deep inspiration and is relieved with sitting up. Dyspnea and radiation to back, epigastrum, or shoulder are sometimes present.

Does the pt have any medical history associated with pericarditis?

Recent myocardial infarction (MI): Can present as soon as 2 to 3 days after an MI.
- Pericarditis presenting much later (several weeks to months) is known as Dressler's syndrome.

Infection (often initially presents as a respiratory infection)
- *Viral*: influenza, varicella, Epstein-Barr virus, coxsackie, echovirus
- *Bacterial*: pneumococcal, streptococcal, staphylococcal, and gonnorheal
- Tuberculosis
- *Fungal*: coccidioidal, candidal

Renal failure: Uremic pericarditis is a common complication in dialysis-dependent pts.

Malignancy: Lung, breast, and renal carcinomas and lymphoma are common causes. Also, the radiation therapy to treat some of these malignancies can lead to pericarditis as well.

Autoimmune: rheumatoid arthritis and systemic lupus erythematosus

Review VS

Low blood pressure, pulsus paradoxus, and rapid heart rate may be the first signs of pericardial effusion causing tamponade, a dangerous complication of pericarditis.

- Tamponade occurs when the pressure exerted by the pericardial fluid exceeds the pressures inside the heart chambers. The atria collapse first, leading to a lack of blood to be ejected by the ventricles. It is a medical emergency and should be treated with immediate pericardiocentesis.

Fever can be seen but is not specific.

Observe the neck veins

Engorged neck veins might suggest pericardial effusion or tamponade physiology.

Auscultate the heart

Friction rub: The classic PE finding is a three-part friction rub.
- Actually sounds like rubbing two pieces of leather together with every beat.

Muffled heart sounds: This is the more common auscultatory finding with pericardial effusion.

Obtain an ECG

Nonspecific ST-T wave changes are common.

Classic findings include ST-segment elevation in all leads (uncommon for an MI), which usually causes ST-segment elevation only in contiguous leads.

Low QRS voltage and electrical alternans may be a sign of effusion.

Obtain a stat CXR

Cardiomegaly may be present from pericardial effusion.

Pericarditis
The pericardium, as the name suggests, is the covering of the heart. It consists of two parts: (1) the visceral pericardium, which sits directly on the heart; and (2) the parietal pericardium, which is a fibrous sac. There is between 15 and 50 mL of pericardial fluid in the sac under normal circumstances. In the case of pericarditis, this amount of fluid is expanded and contains inflammatory cells.
Note the etiology of the pericarditis.
Comment on whether pericardial effusion is present, and if present, if any tamponade physiology is apparent.

Differential diagnosis
Myocardial infarction: substernal chest pain and ECG changes
Pneumonia: pleuritic chest pain
Tension pneumothorax (PTX), restrictive cardiomyopathy, and right ventricular MI can all cause tamponade physiology.
- Tension PTX will be characterized by decreased breath sounds on one side of the chest.

P

An echocardiogram should be urgently ordered if there is any suggestion of pericardial effusion, to assess for the possibility of pericardial tamponade
If tamponade is present, the effusion should be drained by pericardiocentesis or surgically, by pericardial window.

Otherwise, treat the underlying problem
For suspected viral or post-MI pericarditis, start aspirin, up to 900 mg po tid, or another NSAID
After the pt has been afebrile for 7 days, begin to taper the NSAID dose.
If recurrences occur for more than 2 years, refer for pericardectomy.

If you suspect tuberculous pericarditis, perform a purified protein derivative test. If positive, drain pericardial fluid. If no acid-fast bacilli are present and you still suspect TB, biopsy the pericardium for granulomata
If positive, start anti-TB quadruple therapy (INH, rifampin, ethambutol, and pyrazinamide).

For uremic pericarditis, begin daily dialysis for 2 wks. Recheck and perform an echocardiogram at that time
NSAIDs will help relieve symptoms.
If effusion persists after 2 wks, consider drainage.

If the pt has a known malignancy and you suspect neoplastic pericardial effusion, drain the fluid and perform a cytologic study. Consider a partial pericardectomy
Unfortunately, the prognosis for this condition is dismal.

S **Has the pt undergone recent cardiac revascularization (either angioplasty or coronary artery bypass graft) within the last 5 years?**
If so, and the pt does not have any new signs or symptoms of ischemia, further cardiac testing before transferring the pt to the OR is not necessary.

Has the pt had a coronary angiogram or stress test in the last 2 years?
If so, and the results were without evidence of ischemia or infarction, and the pt has no new signs or symptoms of ischemia, further cardiac testing before transferring the pt to the OR is not necessary.

Is there any history of *major* clinical *predictors* of perioperative risk?
- Myocardial infarction (MI)   - Unstable angina
  within the last month   - Severe valvular heart disease
- Decompensated heart failure

Are there any *intermediate* clinical predictors of perioperative risk?
- MI more than 1 month ago   - Stable angina
- Stable congestive heart failure   - Diabetes mellitus
- Renal failure

Are there any *minor* clinical predictors?
History of stroke or poor functional capacity (see below) would be minor clinical predictors.

What is the pt's functional capacity?
Be sure to ask about the pt's ability to walk up a hill or a flight of stairs, wash dishes, or perform light housecleaning duties without dyspnea or chest pain. This question is **crucial** because this represents at least four metabolic equivalents (METs) of activity.

Low functional capacity is < four METs.
- Pts who cannot meet at least four METs because of noncardiac reasons such as severe arthritis should also be labeled as poor functional capacity.

What type of elective surgery is the pt having?
High cardiac risk:
- Emergent major operations in the elderly
- Aortic or other major vascular (except carotid endarterectomy) surgery
- Prolonged surgeries with anticipated blood loss or fluid shifts

Intermediate cardiac risk:
- Carotid endarterectomy   - Head and neck   - Orthopedic
- Intrathoracic   - Intraperitoneal   - Prostate

Low cardiac risk: breast, cataract, endoscopic, and superficial procedures

O **Obtain an ECG, fasting glucose, Hgb A1C, and creatinine. Note age and BP**
Significant arrhythmias such as high-grade atrioventricular block, supraventricular arrhythmias with uncontrolled rate, and symptomatic ventricular arrhythmias in the setting of coronary artery disease are *major* clinical predictors of cardiovascular risk.
Evidence of a prior MI on ECG or diabetes or renal insufficiency (Cr > 2.0) represent *intermediate* clinical predictors of risk.
Advanced age, left ventricular hypertrophy, left bundle branch block, rhythms other than sinus, and hypertension are *minor* predictors of risk.

A —y/o pt with (major/intermediate/minor) predictors of perioperative cardiac events scheduled for (high/intermediate/low) risk surgery

Designate the pt with the highest clinical predictor that you discovered on your evaluation. For example, a pt with three minor clinical predictors and one intermediate clinical predictor is labeled as having an intermediate clinical predictor for perioperative risk for cardiovascular events.

P Refer all pts with major clinical predictors for coronary angiogram before surgery

These pts may require angioplasty or even coronary artery bypass graft before their elective surgery.

If the pt refuses angiogram, he or she should consider delaying or canceling the surgery with medical management and risk factor modification.

Recommend that pts without major but with intermediate clinical predictors with at least MODERATE functional capacity (> 4 METs) can undergo low- to intermediate-risk surgeries without further testing

Their functional capacity indicates that despite their clinical predictors, they likely have enough cardiac function to tolerate one of these surgical procedures.

Refer pts without major but with intermediate predictors with at least MODERATE functional capacity going for high-risk surgeries for noninvasive testing first, such as exercise or pharmacologic stress testing

If noninvasive testing reveals high risk for ischemia, then a coronary angiogram is required, with subsequent care dictated by findings and treatment results.

If noninvasive testing reveals low risk, the pt may proceed to the OR.

Also refer pts without major but with intermediate clinical predictors with LOW functional capacity (< 4 METs) for noninvasive testing

If these tests reveal low risk of ischemia, the pt may proceed to the OR.

If results show high risk, a coronary angiogram is required, with subsequent care dictated by findings and treatment results.

Pts without major or intermediate predictors with at least MODERATE functional capacity may proceed to the OR without further testing

Pts without major or intermediate predictors with LOW functional capacity undergoing high-risk surgeries should undergo noninvasive testing first; for low- or intermediate-risk surgeries, the pt may proceed to the OR without further testing

IV

Gastroenterology

S   Obtain a detailed history regarding the quality and timing of pain

Severe, instantaneous: perforated ulcer, ruptured aneurysm, myocardial infarction
Constant severe pain: acute pancreatitis
Sharp, burning, gnawing, hunger-like pain: peptic ulcer disease (PUD)
Pain that awakens the pt from sleep or 1 to 3 hrs after eating: PUD of the duodenum

What is the relationship between food and pain, if any?

Gastric ulcer, gastroesophageal reflux disease (GERD): worse after food
Duodenal ulcer: tends to be worse before meals

Is there any relief with antacid use?

Duodenal ulcers tend to improve symptomatically after the pt takes antacids.

Is the pt experiencing heartburn or sharp, rising pain in chest?

This type of pain would be typical of GERD.

What medicines is the pt taking? Do they include any NSAIDs?

NSAIDs can cause both duodenal and gastric ulcers.
Antibiotics, especially cyclines, can cause erosive esophagitis.

Ask about any associated symptoms that may raise red flags to rule out cancer

- Family history of cancer
- History of anemia
- Unintentional weight loss
- Hematochezia (bloody stool)
- Feeling of epigastric fullness
- Odynophagia (painful swallowing)
- Hematemesis
- Dysphagia (difficulty swallowing)
- Age older than 45

Any diarrhea, weight loss, or abdominal mass associated with PUD-type symptoms?

This would be consistent with Zollinger-Ellison syndrome, a gastrin-secreting tumor.

Is there any associated nausea or vomiting?

Consider gastric outlet obstruction, which can occur with cancer or chronic PUD.

Is the pt having problems with swallowing? Are liquids easier than solids, or are they the same?

In addition to being symptoms of malignancy, odynophagia and dysphagia may
   indicate an esophageal constriction, ring, web, or achalasia.
- Early mechanical dysphagia will be worse with solids than liquids.
- Advanced mechanical or motor dysphagia creates problems swallowing both.

Has the pt had any prior radiation therapy to the chest?

Radiation can cause esophagitis.

O   Perform a focused PE

Vital signs: Always check BP, heart rate, orthostatics, and temperature.
- Perforated ulcer and pancreatitis may present with tachycardia and unstable vital signs.

Cardiac: Check for tachycardia.
Abd: Make sure the pt does not have a surgical abdomen with rigidity, rebound tenderness, tenderness to percussion, and decreased or absent bowel sounds.
- This may indicate perforated ulcer or pancreatitis.
- PUD may have vague tenderness in the epigastrium or left upper quadrant.

Rectal exam: to rule out bleeding

Check labs
A low hematocrit or positive stool occult blood could be signs of PUD.
If you suspect Zollinger-Ellison syndrome, check the fasting gastrin level (normal
in PUD).

Obtain an upright CXR
This will rule out free air under the diaphragm, which is indicative of perforated ulcer.

Obtain an ECG
To rule out acute coronary syndrome

If the diagnosis is unclear, perform a barium swallow study
This will help diagnose the presence of PUD in up to 80% of cases.

A Epigastric pain
Differential diagnosis includes
Peptic ulcer disease: gastric ulcer, duodenal ulcer, gastric cancer/lymphoma,
   Zollinger-Ellison syndrome (rare), perforation
GERD
Esophagitis: In immunocompromised pt with difficulty swallowing, consider HSV,
   CMV, HIV, or Candida. Can also have radiation-induced or pill esophagitis.
Esophageal strictures, webs, rings, achalasia, or diffuse esophageal spasms
Pancreatitis: Pancreatic inflammation can occur for any number of reasons.
Acute coronary syndrome: Symptoms may be confused with epigastric conditions.

P Pts with the alarm symptoms listed above should undergo immediate
esophagogastroduodenoscopy (EGD)
Best test for malignancy; biopsies performed and other conditions diagnosed visually.

Call an immediate surgery consult for pts with suspected perforated ulcer. For all other pts with ulcers on EGD or suspected ulcers by H&P, start an 8-wk course of a proton pump inhibitor
If after 8 wks symptoms persist, pt should undergo EGD.

Check pts for infection with *Helicobacter pylori*
H. pylori infection is the number one cause of PUD and is extremely common.
The gold standard for diagnosis is histologic exam of antral mucosa via biopsy on EGD.
If not planning EGD, may perform enzyme-linked immunosorbent assay for serum
   IgG against bacterium.
   • If negative, rules out disease. If positive, indicates past exposure, not necessarily
     active disease.
Urease test: *H. pylori* is a urea-splitting organism. Clotest involves the pt swallowing
   radiolabeled urea and then the breath is sampled for radioactive material.
   • Sensitive and specific
   • Pt may not be taking proton pump inhibitor (PPI) before the test.

Treat *H. pylori* if found
Treatment is 2 wks with omeprazole, bismuth, and two antibiotics (varies by regimen).

If you suspect esophageal stricture, the pt will need an EGD
Balloon dilation may be necessary.

Treat all pts with suspected GERD with either a PPI or an H$_2$ blocker
Symptoms should improve on this therapy.

S Ask the pt to describe the pain
Usually pain is epigastric or periumbilical, boring and radiating through to the back. Constant and likely to be relieved a little by leaning forward.

Are there any associated symptoms?
These may include nausea, vomiting, fever, and chills.

Is there any alcohol history?
Especially including the amount consumed and the timing of the last drink. Alcohol is the number one cause of pancreatitis in the United States.

Does the pt have a history of elevated cholesterol?
Hypertriglyceridemia is a risk factor for pancreatitis.

Has the pt had recent abdominal surgery or blunt trauma to the abdomen?
Trauma is also a risk of pancreatitis.

What medicines is the pt taking?
Common medications that may cause pancreatitis include:
- Thiazides   - Sulfonamides   - Cyclines
- Furosemide   - Phenytoin

Has the pt had any symptoms of infection recently?
- Mumps   - Epstein-Barr virus   - Hepatitis A   - Hepatitis B

Has there been any unexplained weight loss?
This symptom should always make you think of cancer.

Is there a history of gallstones?
Gallstones are the most common causes of pancreatitis worldwide.

Has the pt recently had an endoscopic retrograde cholangiopancreaticogram (ERCP)?
Injection of dye into the pancreatic duct may cause pancreatitis.

Is the pt a pregnant or recently pregnant female?
Late in pregnancy, spontaneous pancreatitis may occur.

O Perform a focused PE
Vital signs: Orthostatics, fever, and low oxygen suggest an unstable pt.
Gen: Check for jaundice (a sign of gallstone obstruction).
Abd: Check for presence of bowel sounds and tenderness to palpation/percussion, usually over the epigastrium and periumbilical region.
Skin: Ecchymotic discoloration of the flanks (Grey-Turner's sign) or around the umbilicus (Cullen's sign). Both are associated with a poor prognosis.

Obtain Labs
CBC: Check for increased WBC.
Chemistry: BUN/Cr elevation: Third spacing may compromise renal flow.
- Glucose may be elevated if insulin secretion is impaired.
Cholesterol: Triglyceride level may be elevated.
Check initial amylase and lipase: diagnostic of pancreatitis if elevated.
Hypocalcemia is seen in severe pancreatitis.
Urine pregnancy test
Liver tests: Elevated bilirubin will point to gallstone presence as the cause.
- ALT and LDH elevations are common.

Obtain appropriate imaging studies

Right upper quadrant ultrasound to rule out gallstones and biliary sludge.
CT scan of the abdomen to rule out pancreatic pseudocyst or mass.
CXR: Up to 20% of pts present with left-sided pleural effusions.

Pancreatitis

Pancreatitis is inflammation of the pancreas, worsened by pancreatic enzymes
autodigesting its cellular structure.
As noted from the subjective section, there are many potential causes, including
scorpion sting. It is a potentially lethal condition and should never be taken lightly.
Among the sequelae are decreased pancreatic enzyme production, decreased insulin
production, third spacing of fluid, and acute respiratory distress syndrome.

Keep the pt NPO

Pancreatic rest removes the stimulus to produce more enzymes.
Initiate food when pt is hungry and if no evidence of nausea, vomiting, or ileus is
present.

Relieve pain with meperidine or morphine sulfate

Meperidine is often preferred because other narcotics may cause contraction of the
sphincter of Oddi at the end of the common bile duct.

Replace fluid losses secondary to third spacing

Intravenous hydration with normal saline should be sufficient.
Maintain strict input and output to estimate the amount of fluid sequestered.

If pt becomes unstable, transfer to the ICU. Monitoring and intubation and, rarely, IV antibiotics may be necessary

If pt is not improving, start imipenem to prevent cholangitis or pancreatic abscess.

Consider ERCP if pt has severe pancreatitis or also has cholangitis
Pts with gallstone pancreatitis will need cholecystectomy
Pts with alcohol-induced pancreatitis should abstain from drinking
Treat hyperlipidemia
Place pts with chronic pancreatitis on oral enzyme supplements

Table 4 Ranson's Criteria (predicts morbidity and mortality)	
At the time of admission	**After the initial 48 hours**
Age > 55 years	Decrease in hematocrit > 10%
ALT > 6 × normal	Calcium < 8
LDH > 2 × normal	Increase in BUN > 5
WBC > 16,000	Base deficit > 4
Blood glucose > 200	Estimated fluid sequestration > 600 mL
Arterial pO_2 < 60 mm	

Each index is one point.
The score of 3–4 = 15% mortality; 5–6 = 40% mortality; > 6 = 100% mortality.

S Ask the pt to describe the pain

Sharp, colicky pain in the right upper quadrant, often intermittent, causing the pt to double over in pain; radiating to the shoulder should make you think of gallbladder disease.

Are there any associated symptoms?

Fever: Think acute infectious or inflammatory process
          - Hepatitis   - Cholecystitis   - Ascending cholangitis
Vomiting: obstruction such as gallstone or malignancy
Diarrhea: more common with liver abscess

Is there any relationship of pain with food?

Think of gallstones if pain is worse after fatty meals.

Is the pt an alcohol drinker and has he or she had any alcohol intake recently?

Acute alcoholic hepatitis presents with right upper quadrant (RUQ) pain.

What medications is the pt taking?

Both prescribed and herbal medications may present with drug-induced cholestasis.

Has the pt had any prior surgeries?

Note the reason for surgery and date of surgery.
This will help rule out acute cholecystitis if there has been a cholecystectomy.
It may also point toward a choledocholithiasis (presence of a stone in the common bile duct, retained after the surgery).
Abdominal scars may hurt or cause bowel obstruction secondary to adhesions.

Has there been any recent travel to a third world nation?

Think of hepatitis A

Has the pt had any unintentional weight loss?

This should always make you think of malignancy.

Is there any clay-colored stool or tea-colored urine?

Seen with bilirubin excretion defect

If female, what is the menstrual history?

        - Ovarian torsion   - Ectopic pregnancy
        - Pelvic inflammatory disease   - Endometriosis

Has there been any history of heart disease?

Rarely, cardiac pain can be referred as RUQ pain.

Any cough, chest pain, shortness of breath?

These symptoms indicate a pulmonary or cardiac cause such as:
        - Pneumonia   - Right-sided heart failure   - Pulmonary embolism

O Perform a focused PE

Vital signs: Fever usually indicates infection.
- Tachycardia/orthostatics (as an indirect fluid status assessment)

Gen appearance: jaundice/icterus: gallbladder obstruction, acute hepatitis
Abd: absence of bowel sounds: obstruction; check for ascites.

- *Murphy sign*: inspiratory arrest during light palpation of right hypochondrium: think gallbladder
- Masses palpated, hepatomegaly, splenomegaly
- Jaundice, fever, and RUQ pain: triad indicating ascending cholangitis

Pelvic exam if high suspicion that this may be ovarian in origin
Rectal exam for guaiac test

Obtain these labs

CBC: Presence of elevated WBC suggests infection.
Liver panel to assess for hepatobiliary causes: bilirubin level, transaminases, albumin,
   PT/PTT.
   - AST, ALT > 1000, think acute hepatitis
Check HBsAg, anti-HCV Ab, anti-HAV IgM; if any positive, indicates viral hepatitis.
Amylase elevation > 500 IU suggest pancreatitis, not as specific as elevated lipase level.
Blood cultures: if suspect ascending cholangitis
Pregnancy test
E. histolytica serum titers to rule out amebic liver abscess, if high suspicion

Obtain radiologic studies

RUQ ultrasound: Helps determine the presence of gallstones, gallbladder obstruction,
   gallbladder sludge, as well as liver size, abscesses, or tumors.
Plain film KUB or abdominal film to rule out obstruction
CXR: to rule out pulmonary causes
CT of abdomen may be needed for pancreatic evaluation, liver abscesses
HIDA scan: if you suspect acute cholecystitis, cystic duct obstruction

A **Right upper quadrant pain**
Differential diagnosis includes

Gallbladder diseases: acute cholecystitis, ascending cholangitis, common bile duct
   stone, gallbladder cancer (cholangiocarcinoma)
Liver diseases: hepatitis (alcoholic/viral), abscesses, tumors
Pancreas: gallstone pancreatitis, pancreatic pseudocyst, pancreatic carcinoma
Pulm: pneumonia, pulmonary embolism
Cardiac: right-sided failure with passive hepatic congestion (nutmeg liver on
   pathology)
Bowel obstruction
Pelvic: ovarian torsion, ectopic pregnancy, pelvic inflammatory disease, endometriosis

P **Begin with supportive care**

Narcotics for pain control
IV hydration with normal saline

Call surgery if pt has acute abdomen or signs of obstruction

These include decreased bowel sounds, rigidity, guarding, and tenderness to percussion.

Treat based on the underlying disorder

Cholecystectomy is the treatment for acute cholecystitis/choledocholithiasis and
   gallstone pancreatitis. Consider prophylactic antibiotics.
   - May need medical stabilization before treatment with nasogastric suctioning and
      volume resuscitation.
Acute hepatitis: supportive care, may need ICU monitoring
Liver abscess (pyogenic or amebic): antibiotics
   - Consider drainage if pt has persistent fever or unclear diagnosis.
Ascending cholangitis: antibiotics; endoscopic retrograde cholangiopancreatography
   or percutaneous drainage may be required. Asymptomatic or intermittently painful
   gallstone disease does not require surgery.

S **Does the pt have any other symptoms of biliary disease?**
  - Yellow eyes   - Itchiness   - Dark urine and light-colored stool

Are there any risk factors for hepatitis?
  - IV drug abuse   - Needle sharing   - Unprotected sex
  - Tattoos   - Blood transfusions (prior surgeries, especially
                       before 1982)

What medications is the pt taking?
  - Tylenol   - Antiepileptics   - Lipid-lowering medications

Does the pt drink alcohol?
Ask about duration and amount.

Has the pt traveled to or emigrated from a third world nation?
  - Viral hepatitides   - Yellow fever
  - Malaria   - Entamoebic diseases

Has there been any recent unexplained weight change?
Unintentional weight loss should lead you to think of cancer.
Rapid weight gain may indicate development of ascites.

Does the pt have diabetes, high cholesterol, and/or obesity?
These conditions are risk factors for nonalcoholic fatty liver disease (NAFLD).

Is there any family history of liver disease?
Both hemachromatosis (a disease of iron overload) and Wilson's disease (copper
  overload) are genetic causes of abnormal liver tests.

Does the pt have a history of any autoimmune disease?
Autoimmune diseases can cause autoimmune hepatitis or primary biliary cirrhosis.

O **Check the VS**
Fever, hypotension, tachycardia: infectious hepatic process or end-stage liver disease

Physical evidence of liver disease on the general exam includes
  - Jaundice   - Telangectasias
  - White nail beds   - Gynecomastia

Signs of liver disease on the abdominal exam include
  - Flank dullness   - Ascites   - Hepatomegaly
  - Splenomegaly   - Right upper quadrant tenderness

**Send blood for liver function tests, viral hepatits panel, an antinuclear
antibody (ANA) and an anti-smooth muscle antibody (ASMA), serum
iron studies, α_1-antitrypsin level, and a serum ceruloplasmin level**
Albumin: Many illnesses can affect the liver's production of albumin, but in the
  presence of known liver disease, this is evidence that function has been affected.
Prothrombin time (PT): The liver produces many of the coagulation factors. When
  production is affected, PT increases.
Bilirubin: Cholestatic disease presents with an elevation of direct and total bilirubin.
Alanine aminotransferase (ALT): specific for liver, muscle
Aspartate aminotransferase (AST): present in liver, heart muscle, kidney, brain, and red
  blood cells
  • Moderately elevated enzymes, AST > ALT by > 2:1, consider alcoholic hepatitis
  • Otherwise, ALT will usually be > AST.
Alkaline phosphatase (AP): produced in biliary ducts, bone, placenta, and intestines

- Extrahepatic sources of elevated AP can be differentiated from hepatic by a normal 5'nucleosidase level. It will be elevated with liver disease.

Viral hepatitis panel: Consider anti-HAV IgM, HbsAg, anti-HBc, and anti-HCV as primary tests for active liver disease to rule out hepatitis A, B, and C. See Hepatitis, p. 58.

ANA and ASMA: One or the other should be positive in autoimmune hepatitis.

Ferritin, iron, and iron saturation will all be markedly elevated in the presence of hemachromatosis, which usually presents in the fifth decade of life.

Ceruloplasmin will be elevated in Wilson's disease, which usually presents late in the second decade or early in the third decade of life.

α_1-antitrypsin will be low in its deficiency; another inherited cause of liver disease.

Obtain an ultrasound of the right upper quadrant
Diagnoses presence of gallstones, masses, obstruction, abscesses, or cirrhosis.

Liver disease
Decide if this is hepatocellular injury versus a cholestatic picture.
- ↑↑↑ AST/ALT with ↑ AP and total bilirubin, think hepatocellular injury.
- ↑↑↑ Total bilirubin, AP elevation with ± AST/ALT elevation, think cholestasis.

Differential diagnosis of hepatocellular injury
Viral hepatitis: A, B, C, D, E, CMV, EBV, HSV, VZV
Autoimmune hepatitis
NAFLD: Fatty degeneration of hepatocytes occurs with metabolic syndrome as noted above.
Toxic hepatitis: acetaminophen, alcohol, other medications and toxins
Vascular causes: Budd-Chiari (hepatic vein thrombosis), congestive heart failure, shock liver
Hereditary causes: hemochromatosis, α_1-antitrypsin deficiency, Wilson's disease

Differential diagnosis of cholestatic injury
Obstructive: choledocholithiasis, cholangiocarcinoma, pancreatic cancer, sclerosing cholangitis
Nonobstructive: cirrhosis, sepsis, postoperative, primary biliary cirrhosis

For most liver diseases, pts will require supportive care and close observation
Viral hepatitides may improve spontaneously. If they become chronic, refer to hepatology.
For autoimmune hepatitis, give steroids and other immunosuppressive agents as indicated.
For NAFLD, encourage the pt to lose weight. This may reverse some of the damage.
For obstructive lesions, refer pt to a surgeon or gastroenterologist to relieve the lesions.

For pts with cirrhosis or genetic lesions that will cause cirrhosis, consider transplant
Unfortunately, placing a pt on the transplant list may be all that can be done.

Give Vitamin K for pts with elevated PT/PTT
This may improve production of clotting factors.

All pts with elevated liver enzymes should be instructed to refrain from alcohol
Repeat abnormal liver tests every 6 months. If no diagnosis is evident, pt may need biopsy

S **Is the pt having any symptoms commonly associated with hepatitis?**
- Jaundice   - Itching   - Fatigue
- Fevers   - Right upper quadrant pain   - Vomiting/diarrhea

Are there any risk factors for hepatitis?
- Blood transfusions   - IV drug use   - Tattoos
- Unprotected sex   - Cocaine use

Does the pt have a history of hepatitis in the past?
A history of hepatitis B puts the pt at risk for infection with hepatitis D (Delta).

Has the pt received any vaccinations for a hepatitis virus?
Hepatitis B is vaccinated against at birth, with a three-shot series (birth, 1 month, and 6 months).
Hepatitis A vaccine is started at age 2 years with a booster after 6 months.

Does the pt have a history of any autoimmune diseases?
These may put the pt at risk for autoimmune hepatitis and primary biliary cirrhosis.
- Commonly occurs in women ages 30 to 65 and can occur without prior autoimmune diseases.

Has the pt recently consumed alcohol?
Acute alcoholic hepatitis can be severe.

Is the pt from, or has he or she recently traveled to, a third world nation?
Although viral hepatitides are common in the United States, they are even more common in the third world.

Is the pt taking or receiving any medications?
Toxic hepatitis is common. Consider acetaminophen, isoniazid, niacin, and phenytoin.

O **Perform a thorough PE**
Vital signs: if ↓ BP, ↑ HR, consider fulminant hepatic failure.
- Fever is more likely in acute hepatitis A and E.
Eyes: icteric sclerae
Neck: Cervical lymphadenopathy may occur.
Abd: Liver is usually enlarged and tender to palpation.
- Splenomegaly may occur.
Skin: jaundice; rarely, pts will have spider angiomata.

Serum markers for hepatitis are imperative for making the diagnosis
Anti-HAV: IgM (+) indicates current infection; IgG (+) indicates previous infection.
HbsAg: The presence of hepatitis B surface antigen indicates ongoing active infection.
If it is negative, the pt does not have active hepatitis B.
Anti-HBc: IgM (+) indicates acute infection; IgG (+) indicates previous infection if surface antigen negative, chronic infection if surface antigen positive.
Anti-HCV: Rarely found in the acute phase because generally asymptomatic.
Therefore, only necessary to test IgG. If positive, HCV infection can be assumed.
Far more rarely:
- Anti-HDV: If co-infecting with HBV, anti-HBc IgM will be positive; if superinfecting a pt who already has HBV, anti-HBc IgG will be positive.
- Anti-HEV: as with anti-HAV

Check markers of hepatocyte inflammation

Alanine aminotransferase (ALT): specific for liver, muscle

Aspartate aminotransferase (AST): present in liver, heart muscle, kidney, brain, and red
blood cells

- Moderately elevated enzymes, AST > ALT by ≥ 2:1, consider alcoholic hepatitis.
- Otherwise, ALT will usually be > AST.
- If elevations mild, consider chronic hepatitis (see Abnormal Liver Tests, p. 56).

Total bilirubin: commonly 5–20 mg/dL

Prothrombin time (PT): Clotting factors are made by the liver. Prolongation suggests a
severe defect in protein synthesis; may indicate a worse prognosis.

Antinuclear antibody, anti-LKM, anti-SMA: May indicate autoimmune hepatitis.

 Hepatitis

Any syndrome causing inflammation of the liver. Can be acute or chronic.

Differential diagnosis of acute hepatitis

- Hepatitis A	- Hepatitis B	- Hepatitis D
- Hepatitis E	- Alcoholic	- Toxic

Differential diagnosis of chronic hepatitis

- Hepatitis B	- Hepatitis C	- Autoimmune hepatitis

Key points with regard to these diagnoses

Both hepatitis A and E are transmitted by the fecal–oral route. Incubation is
approximately 4 wks, and fecal shedding occurs before clinical symptoms. If there is
not an outbreak or a concentration in a home, it is unlikely that you will find the
source.

Hepatitis B causes chronic hepatitis in a minority of cases but is more common with
younger age of infection. Maternal–infant transmission, sexual contact, and IV drug
abuse are most common.

Hepatitis C is rarely transmitted via the sexual route. Usually tattoos, snorting cocaine,
IV drug usage, and blood transfusion (not screened for until the late 1980s) are most
common.

P **Hospitalize only for inability to tolerate oral intake or if you suspect
fulminant hepatitis**

For acute viral hepatitis, there is no effective treatment. Supportive care is most
important.

If the pt has autoimmune hepatitis, consider steroids.

Discharge when PT begins to improve or pt can tolerate oral intake.

- Consider vitamin K IM or SQ to enhance coagulase production.

For fulminant hepatitis, consider ICU monitoring

Only in the ICU will you be able to follow the shifting fluids and electrolytes and treat
all of the possible complications. Liver transplant will likely be necessary.

For pts with chronic hepatitis, advise them to refrain from alcohol consumption

Alcohol greatly increases the risk of hepatocellular carcinoma in these pts.

Check liver tests, α-fetal protein, and ultrasound every 6 months to monitor for cirrhosis or malignancy. Refer pts with HBV or HCV to hepatology

Interferon therapy may be effective in these pts. Consider transplant for cirrhotics.

S   Does the pt have any history of drinking alcohol?
Ask about the amount of alcohol consumption: how much for how many years.

Is there a family history of liver cirrhosis?
Genetic causes: hemochromatosis, Wilson's disease, α_1-antitrypsin deficiency

Has the pt had increased itching?
Increased bilirubin tends to cause itching but is also the presenting sign of primary biliary cirrhosis.

Does the pt take oral contraceptives or is there a history of a hypercoaguable state?
Hypercoagulability and oral contraceptive use are risk factors for Budd Chiari, a hepatic vein thrombosis.

Ask about more unusual potential diagnoses
Hemochromotosis: Suspect in a pt with diabetes, bronze skin, and hypogonadism.
Wilson's disease: Suspect in a young pt with neurologic or psychiatric disease.

O   Perform a generalized PE
Vital signs:
- *Low BP*: increased third spacing of fluid
- *Fever*: spontaneous bacterial peritonitis

Gen: Look for gynecomastia, fetor hepaticus, and bilateral parotid enlargement.
Neuro: Assess mental status to determine if hepatic encephalopathy is present.
- If pt seems altered, have pt hold arms out in front of body, hyperextended at the wrists. If hepatic encephalopathy is present, hands will flap down and back up again; known as asterixis.

Skin: Look for spider angiomas, jaundice, and palmar erythema, all signs of cirrhosis.
Eyes: Conjunctival icterus is the first sign of jaundice.
- If you suspect Wilson's disease, look for a Kayser-Fleischer ring in the iris.

Abd:
- *Ascites*: flank dullness, fullness, distention; check for fluid wave or shifting dullness.
- *Caput medusae*: visible veins on surface of abdomen, surrounding umbilicus
- *Hepatosplenomegaly*: Splenomegaly is more common because of portal venous. congestion. Cirrhotic livers are usually small/shrunken. Hepatomegaly may indicate malignancy.

Testicles: Check for atrophy.

Perform lab analyses to aid in diagnosis
Transaminases (AST/ALT): Elevation implies ongoing hepatocellular destruction.
Hepatitis B surface antigen: If positive, indicates active hepatitis B infection.
Hepatitis C antibody: If positive, assume that pt has ongoing chronic hepatitis C.
Cerulosplasmin: If elevated, the pt has Wilson's.
Iron panel: Elevated ferritin and iron saturation may indicate hemochromatosis.
α_1-*antitrypsin*: Low level indicates deficiency syndrome.
Antimitochondrial antibody: Indicates primary biliary cirrhosis.
Alpha fetal protein: If elevated, may indicate occult hepatocellular carcinoma (HCC).

Follow-up with lab analyses to aid in management
CBC: Cirrhosis is associated with anemia, leukopenia, and thrombocytopenia.
Chemistry: ↓ Na^+ secondary to ascites; elevated NH_3 may indicate encephalopathy.

Obtain a right upper quadrant (RUQ) ultrasound
Detects ascites, cirrhosis, hepatic masses, hepatic/portal vein patency, and biliary
   dilation.

If unsure of diagnosis, obtain a liver biopsy
This is the gold standard for the diagnosis of cirrhosis, usually done percutaneously.

Cirrhosis
Assess for the Child-Pugh Score: A = 5–6; B = 7–9; C = 10–15. Lower number: better
   outcome (Table 5).

P **All cirrhotics should avoid alcohol. If etiology is known, treat the
underlying disorder**
Phlebotomy for hematochromatosis; d-penicillamine for Wilson's disease
Give antiviral agents such as interferon alpha and ribavarin for viral hepatitis.

**If ascites is present, perform a paracentesis to rule out spontaneous
bacterial peritonitis (SBP)**
Send fluid for cell count and differential, albumin, consider total protein LDH, and
   glucose.
Treat with IV Cefepime for SBP if PMN > 250 cells/mm or if neutrophil > 50% of cells.

Obtain a serum ascites albumin gradient
Subtract ascitic albumin from serum albumin. If > 1.1, the pt has portal hypertension.

Restrict dietary sodium to less than 2 g or 88 mmol per day
This should decrease ascites development.
Fluid restriction is not necessary unless the pt is severely hyponatremic.

Give oral diuretics if ascites is present
Furosemide 40 mg orally qd and spironolactone 100 mg qd. Always in a 5:2 ratio.

Give lactulose, titrating to three bowel movements per day
Increased clearance of colonic flora should reduce encephalopathy.

**Place the pt on the list to be evaluated for a liver transplant
Screen for HCC q 6 months with RUQ ultrasound and serum alpha
fetal protein**

Table 5 Child-Pugh Score			
	1	2	3
Ascites	none	slight	moderate/severe
Encephalopathy	none	slight	moderate/severe
Bilirubin (mg/dL)	< 2	2–3	> 3
Albumin (mg/L)	> 3.5	2.8–3.5	< 2.8
PT (seconds increased)	1–3	4–6	> 6

S How large are the bowel movements? What is the consistency of the stool?

Voluminous/watery: Implies small bowel/proximal colon source, osmotic diarrhea.
 • Pt is more likely to have electrolyte imbalances.
Small: Think left colon or rectum.

What are the associated symptoms?
Inflammatory: pain, tenesmus, fever
Osmotic: cramps, bloating, flatulence

What did the pt eat recently? What does he or she eat regularly?
Preformed bacterial toxicities can come from consuming expired milk products, mayonnaise, or old fried rice. These include *Staphylococcus aureus and Bacillus cereus*.
Fruit or milk products may aggravate diarrhea. Fructose or lactose intolerance are common.

Does fasting improve the diarrhea?
Osmotic diarrhea stops with fasting, whereas secretory diarrhea will continue.

Is there blood in the stool?
If bloody diarrhea, always think of colitis, infectious versus inflammatory.
Other etiologies of bloody stool (although usually will not be diarrhea) are hemorrhoids, colonic malignancy, arterial malformations, and venous mesenteric thrombosis.

Is the stool foul smelling or greasy in appearance?
If there is visible oil, this is known as steattorhea. It is caused by malabsorption.

What medications has the pt been taking?
Antibiotic usage puts the pt at risk for diarrhea or even *Clostridium difficile* colitis.

Has the pt recently traveled abroad or gone camping?
Travel abroad puts the pt at risk for parasitic infections.
Drinking from stream water is a risk for *Giardia lamblia*, a small intestinal parasite.

 Perform a focused PE
Vital signs: Presence of fever could point to infectious or inflammatory causes.
 • A pt with positive orthostatic blood pressure or pulse is hypovolemic.
Gen appearance: Look for rashes, mouth ulcers, flushing, or any other systemic signs.
Abd: Usually nonspecific tenderness, but check for bowel sounds.
Rectal: Check for tone, presence of perianal fistulas/abscesses.

Check stool analyses
| - WBC | - Occult blood | - Fat | - Culture |
| - pH | - Laxatives | - O & P | - *C. difficile* toxin |

Check stool electrolytes and calculate a stool osmotic gap.
 • The osmotic gap is $290-2(Na + K)$ mOsmol/kg.
 • In pure osmotic diarrhea, the gap is greater than 125.

Consider other labs for suspected diagnoses
Urine for 5-hydroxyindole acid, the metabolite of serotonin, is the test for carcinoid.
For malabsorption, send serum for antigliadin and antiendomysial (tests for celiac sprue).

Diarrhea

Defined as greater than 200 g/day of stool; average daily output is 150–180 g/day. Acute diarrhea is of less than 2 wks, whereas chronic is greater than 2 to 3 wks.

Differential diagnosis of acute diarrhea. Most are infectious

Enterotoxic: These are secretory diarrheas of the small intestine. Occult blood/WBCs are negative.

- Bacterial: *Vibrio cholera* and most types of *Escherichia coli*
- Viral: Rotavirus, Norvovirus (previously called Norwalk agent)
- Parasitic: *Giardia lamblia*

Invasive: These are inflammatory diarrheas. Occult blood/WBCs are positive.

- Bacterial: *Campylobacter jejuni*, Salmonella, Shigella, *E. coli* O157:H7, *C. difficile*, etc.
- Parasitic: *Entamoeba histolytica*, tapeworm infections

Pts with AIDS may not have fever. Organisms include Cryptosporidia, *E. histolytica*, Giardia, Isospora, Strongyloides, Mycobacterium, cytomegalovirus, etc. Likely if CD4 count < 200.

Inflammatory bowel diseases (IBD), ulcerative colitis, Crohn's disease can present acutely.

Differential diagnosis of chronic diarrhea

Osmotic diarrheas: Those in which molecules create osmotic load, pulling water into stool.

- Celiac sprue	- Intestinal lymphoma	- Bacterial overgrowth
- Drug-induced	- Pancreatic insufficiency	- Lactose intolerance
- Short gut syndrome		

Secretory diarrheas: Water and electrolytes are secreted into the stool.

- Carcinoid	- Zollinger-Ellison	- VIP-oma

Inflammatory diarrheas: Noninfectious causes are fairly limited to IBD.

Intestinal wall motion can also be altered. This includes pheochromocytoma, hyperthyroidism, and irritable bowel syndrome.

AIDS enteropathy should always be considered in the differential of chronic diarrhea.

If the pt is dehydrated, admit and begin IV fluid/electrolyte replacement

Then determine the cause of diarrhea and treat accordingly

Acute: For most acute forms of diarrhea, watchful waiting will be all that is indicated. If risk factors indicate, pts may need sigmoidoscopy to rule out ischemia or ulcers.

For chronic diarrheas, start oral loperamide as the cause is investigated

Loperamide decreases intestinal motility. For investigation, consider colonoscopy.

For osmotic diarrheas, dietary changes and oral enzyme therapy may improve symptoms

For IBD, immunosuppressants and NSAIDs, orally and as enemas, should decrease ulcers

If a parasitic infection is detected on the stool ova and parasite study, give specific therapy

S **Is the pt vomiting bright red blood or something that looks like coffee grounds?**

This will help determine the acuity of the situation. Blood that has been in the stomach for a while will look like coffee grounds secondary to the effects of gastric enzymes.

Ask the pt to describe the amount of blood seen and events leading to the bleeding.

Did vomiting/retching precede the bleeding?

Emesis or retching raises intraesophageal pressure.

Multiple normal emeses or retches before actually vomiting blood implies a tear of the esophagus, also known as a Mallory-Weiss tear.

Has the pt had any associated symptoms, such as fatigue, dyspnea, or chest pain?

These symptoms suggest that severe anemia has been long-standing.

Does the pt have any risk factors for gastric or duodenal erosions?

These include use of nonsteroidal anti-inflammatory drugs (NSAIDs), cigarette smoking, alcohol usage (risk of liver disease and esophageal varices), and recent trauma/central nervous system injury/or burns, usually followed by an ICU stay.

Has the pt vomited blood in the past?

It is very common with decompensated liver disease that pts will have multiple episodes of esophageal varices that need banding.

Has the pt had any black, tarry, foul-smelling stools?

Black stool is likely melena or digested blood appearing as stool.

It is a sign of an upper GI bleed because the digestion process occurs in the small intestine.

Has the pt had any frankly bloody stool?

Bloody stool could represent colonic/rectal bleeding (most likely), but a significantly brisk upper GI bleed can pass through the small intestine fast enough to avoid digestion.

- In that case, the pt should appear unstable; see below.

Was the pt actually vomiting, or did the blood come up with coughing?

It is important to differentiate between hematemesis versus hemoptysis.

Has the pt had a recent nosebleed and, if so, how did he or she stop it?

Many people stop nosebleeds by holding their heads back. Blood runs into the stomach. It is a gastric irritant and a potent emetic. Subsequent hematemesis is common.

O **If the pt is actively having hematemesis, perform a rapid, focused PE**

Vital signs: Increased pulse, decreased blood pressure, and positive orthostatics are all emergent signs indicating that the pt will need volume resuscitation.

Gen apprearance:
- *Pale conjuctivae, poor skin turgor*: suggests anemia
- *Spider angiomas, jaundice*: suggests portal hypertension; think of esophageal varices.

Cardiac: Look for tachycardia, high-output flow murmur implying anemia.

Abd: bowel sounds, ascites, hepatosplenomegaly

Rectal exam is a must to determine the presence of brisk bleeding.

Check labs

Check the CBC: Hgb may be normal, but it takes 2 hrs of bleeding to decrease 25%;

50% is seen at 8 hrs, and the final equilibrated number will not be noted until 72 hrs.
- Platelets are often elevated with a GI bleed, or they may be low in the case of cirrhosis.

Check BUN/Cr: BUN may be elevated in a GI bleed.

Also check liver function tests (bilirubin, albumin, PT/PTT). High bilirubins, prolonged clotting times, and low albumin are all associated with chronic liver disease.

Upper gastrointestinal bleed
Differential diagnosis includes

Peptic ulcer disease: Ulcers can occur in either the stomach or the duodenum. Most common etiologies include *Helicobacter pylori* infection, NSAID use, and smoking.

Gastric erosions: Can occur secondary to pills or stress, possibly in an ICU setting.

Esophagitis: Inflammation of the esophagus can cause slow bleeding.

Esophageal varices: In the setting of cirrhosis, portal venous pressure increases. When this is elevated, those veins that anastamose with systemic venous circulation can become swollen. In this setting, rupture and brisk bleeding are likely.

Mallory-Weiss tear: See above. Can make diagnosis clinically or on endoscopy.

GI malignancy: Cancer in any portion of the GI tract can cause GI bleeding. Rarely brisk.

Hemorrhoids or diverticulosis: Bright red blood per rectum in a stable pt with a relatively normal hemoglobin is likely to have a perirectal cause.

Findings on esophagogastroduodenoscopy (EGD) and risk of rebleeding
Clean-based ulcer: 5%
Red dot ulcer base: 10%
Adherent clot: 20% to 30%
Visible vessel: 50%
Spurting vessel: 90%

For unstable pts, resuscitate with crystalloid (normal saline or Ringer's lactate)

Volume resuscitation is the first and most important step in the treatment of acute GI bleed!

Transfuse pt with packed red blood cells
Goal hematocrit should be ≥ 30.

Pt will require IV access with a large-bore catheter to ensure rapid transfusion and crystalloid infusion. Consider placing a central line.
- May need fresh frozen plasma if still bleeding and increased PT.

Place a nasogastric tube
This will help determine whether the pt is still actively bleeding.

Also serves as the way to clear the stomach before EGD.

Call an emergent GI consult
This pt requires an emergent EGD.

Once bleeding has ceased
Pt will need a proton pump inhibitor upon discharge.

If bleeding is caused by esophageal varices, consider β-blockers and repeat EGD as per GI.

Pt may be discharged home if clean-based ulcer, nonbleeding ulcer, mild gastritis, or low-grade esophagitis.

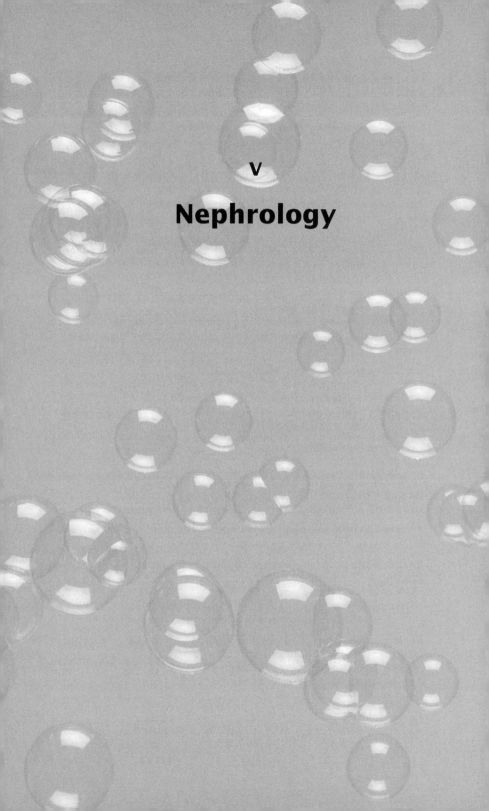

V

Nephrology

S   Does the pt have a known history of hypertension (HTN)?

If so, note the age of onset and what previous medications were used to treat it.
Ask if there is a family history of HTN, cardiovascular disease, or strokes.

Does the pt take anything associated with HTN?

These would include alcohol, cocaine, high daily salt intake, cigarette smoking, oral
contraceptives, NSAIDs, steroids, or decongestants.

Does the pt have symptoms that suggest secondary causes of HTN?

Renovascular HTN: abrupt onset in < 30 y/o, difficult to control with medicine
Primary aldosteronism: muscle weakness and cramps, and periodic paralysis
Pheochromocytoma: episodic headaches, hypertensive episodes, diaphoresis,
palpitations, and weight loss

Does pt report any risk factors associated with poorer prognosis?

- Smoking   - Sedentary   - Obesity
- Dyslipidemia   - Diabetes mellitus

O   What is the pt's blood pressure?

Obtain at least two blood pressure (BP) measurements with the pt in the supine or
seated position. Each measurement should be at least 2 to 3 minutes apart. Meaure in
both arms and use the highest value.

Look for evidence of end-organ damage

- Left ventricular hypertrophy   - Myocardial infarction
- Congestive heart failure   - Papilledema
- Renal insufficiency   - Stroke
- Retinal exudates

Perform a fundoscopic exam

This exam offers a rare opportunity to directly visualize arteries and veins.
Look for atrioventricular nicking, arterial narrowing, retinal exudates, or hemorrhages.

Examine the heart

Look for S_4, ventricular lift, murmurs, and a loud aortic component of S_2.

Perform a complete neurologic assessment

HTN can cause both ischemic or hemorrhagic strokes.

Examine the pt for any signs of secondary HTN

Renovascular HTN: abdominal bruit
Cushing syndrome: edema, striae of abdomen
Hyperthyroidism: enlarged thyroid gland, exophthalmos
Coarctation of the aorta: diminished/delayed femoral > upper extremity pulses

Perform urine and blood tests to screen for secondary causes of HTN or increased risk of poor outcomes

Primary aldosteronism: low potassium and high sodium
Renovascular disease: elevated BUN, creatinine, and proteinuria
Poorer prognosis: diabetes (especially if not well controlled) and dyslipidemia

Perform an ECG

Look for evidence of chronic HTN (left ventricular hypertrophy) and evidence of old
infarctions (q waves).

A **Hypertension**
Blood pressure measured above the normal range on three separate occasions.
Attempt to identify the cause of the hypertension:
- Most cases (90%) are labeled essential, meaning the cause is unknown.
- Secondary causes are usually either renal (5%) or endocrine (4%).
Assign the pt to the higher category if diastolic and systolic values fall in different categories (Table 6).

P **Start drug therapy on any pt with at least high normal HTN or greater with target organ disease or cardiovascular disease and/or diabetes**
Diruetics: uncomplicated hypertension, heart failure, type 2 diabetes
β-blockers: uncomplicated hypertension, myocardial infarction, angina, atrial fibrillation, essential tremor, hyperthyroidism, preoperative HTN
ACE inhibitor: diabetes with proteinuria, heart failure, myocardial infarction with systolic dysfunction
Calcium channel blockers: type 1 and 2 diabetes with proteinuria
Non-DHP calcium channel blockers: isolated systolic hypertension in elderly, migraine headache, atrial tachycardia or fibrillation
α-*blocker*: benign prostatic hypertrophy

Encourage lifestyle modifications in pts with high normal BP who do not have diabetes, target organ disease, or cardiovascular disease but have none or one risk factor
- Weight loss   - < 1 oz alcohol/day ethanol   - < 2.4 g sodium
- ↓ fats   - Smoking cessation   - Aerobic exercise 30 min/day

Any pt with stage I HTN with no risk factors or any target organ or cerebrovascular disease should have a trial of 12 months of lifestyle modification
If pt has only one risk factor that is not diabetes, try lifestyle modifications for only 6 months.
If BP is not normal at the end of this period, initiate drug therapy.

Start drug therapy in any pt with stage 2 or 3 HTN
Attempt to rule out secondary causes of hypertension
Renovascular HTN: captopril stimulation test of plasma renin activity
Primary aldosteronism: 24-hr urinary aldosterone collection
Pheochromocytoma: urinary test for VMA, metanephrins, and catecholamines
Cushing syndrome: 24-hr collection of urinary free cortisol or overnight dexamethasone suppression test

Table 6 Hypertension Categories		
Category	**Systolic (mm Hg)**	**Diastolic (mm Hg)**
Normal	< 120	< 80
Prehypertension	130–139	85–89
Stage I	140–159	90–99
Stage II	> 160	> 100

S

Does the pt report any swelling or edema?
With oliguria there is often a buildup of fluid in the soft tissues, manifesting as edema in dependent areas such as the ankles and, if supine, the presacral area.

Has the pt had decreased urine output?
As urine output drops, monitor the pt carefully and dialyze when indicated.

Any confusion, malaise, muscle cramps, or weakness?
These are very common symptoms in acute renal failure.

Does the pt have any heart, liver, or kidney disease?
Cardiovascular conditions such as CHF can cause a prerenal insult and provoke ARF.
Liver conditions such as hemochromatosis and autoimmune hepatitis are commonly associated with renal disease.
Pts with autosomal-dominant polycytic kidney disease will have cysts in the liver and atrioventricular malformations in the brain.

Does the pt have a history of kidney stones?
Bilateral kidney stones are a rare cause of ARF.

Does the pt have any history of vomiting, diarrhea, or other volume loss?
Volume depletion from the GI tract or the kidneys can cause ARF.

Is the pt taking any nephrotoxic drugs?
Antibiotics: aminoglycosides, amphotericin, pentamidine, vancomycin
Chemotherapeutics: cisplatin, cyclosporin, ifosfamide
Anesthesia: nitrous oxide, isoflurane
Anticholinergics, such as TCAs, can cause obstructive ARF.

Has the pt had any IV contrast for imaging lately?
Increased risk of renal failure in pts suffering from chronic illnesses such as diabetes mellitus, CHF, and HTN. Creatinine (Cr) rises within 48 hrs of insult.

O

Review VS and perform a full PE, specifically including
HTN and fluid overload are common in glomerulonephritis (GN).
Hypotension and tachycardia suggest hypovolemia.
Gen: Assess mental status.
Neck: Elevated jugular venous distention indicates fluid overload.
Cardio: S_3/S_4 gallops/murmur suggest heart failure; rubs suggest pericarditis.
Pulm: Crackles suggest fluid overload.
Ext: Edema
Skin: Pallor and ecchymoses. Rash may indicate AIN.

Order strict I/Os and review the numbers
To differentiate between oliguric (< 400 mL/day) and nonoliguric renal failure

Check BUN/Cr
Elevated ratio of BUN to Cr > 20:1 is seen in prerenal causes.
Elevated Cr represents renal failure. (It takes a loss of about 90% of renal function to double Cr.) Creatinine is dependent on muscle mass of pt:
- Thin, nonmuscular woman can be as low as 0.6; 70-kg man should be about 0.9.
- Very muscular men can get up around 1.2.
- So Cr 1.2 in a small woman is considered renal failure.

Check serum electrolytes
K and Phos are high. HCO_3 and Ca are low.
In chronic renal failure, the electrolyte abnormalities are less pronounced.

Review the pt's CBC
The kidneys produce erythropoietin, which is needed for RBC production.
In renal failure, especially if chronic, anemia is common; less likely in acute.
Eosinophilia suggests acute interstitial nephritis.

Review urinalysis
- *Hematuria*: nephritis or infection   - *Proteinuria*: nephrotic syndrome
- *WBC casts*: AIN   - *RBC casts*: glomerulonephritis
- *Granular casts*: ATN   - *Eosinophiluria*: AIN

Calculate a Fractional Excretion of Sodium (FE$_{Na}$)
$FE_{Na} = Urine_{Na}/Plasma_{Na} \times Plasma_{Cr}/Urine_{Cr} \times 100$ (unreliable s/p diuretics).
- If $FE_{Na} < 1$ consider prerenal   • If $FE_{Na} > 2$ intrinsic/postrenal

Obtain a renal ultrasound
Look for small (< 10 cm), scarred (chronic renal failure), polycystic, hydronephrosis
(obstruction), or other abnormalities of the kidney.

Obtain postvoid residual to rule out obstruction
Foley catheter inserted after void. Amount of urine should be < 25 mL.

Acute Renal Failure
Loss of significant renal function over a relatively short period of time.

Etiologies
Prerenal: volume depletion, excessive vasodilation or vasoconstriction
Renal: parenchymal disease
- ATN: The two main causes of ATN are ischemia and toxic injury.
  - ◆ Renal ischemia: hypovolemia, sepsis, CHF, cyclosporine
  - ◆ Endogenous toxin: myoglobin, calcium, myeloma light-chain
  - ◆ Exogenous toxin: IV contrast, aminoglycosides
- GN: RBC casts on U/A have multiple possible etiologies, such as:
  - Poststreptococcal GN   - IgA nephropathy
  - Membranoproliferative GN   - Rapidly progressive GN
  - Vasculitis: Wegener's granulomatosis, Henoch-Schönlein purpura
- AIN: characterized by renal failure, fever, eosinophilia, and rash
  - ◆ Caused by medications such as Bactrim, allopurinol, and NSAIDs.
Postrenal: ureteral (bilateral ureteral stones), bladder, or uretheral obstruction
(enlarged prostate, TCA, or other drugs with anticholinergic effects)

If prerenal due to hypovolemia, nonoliguric, replace with normal saline
Boluses 20 cc/kg, then run infusion at 150 to 200 mL/hr (slower if decreased cardiac
function, preexisting renal disease, or elderly).

Monitor fluid status by strict I/O, vital signs, and daily weights
Ensure adequate urine output to avoid volume overload in these pts.

Treat ATN and rhabdomyolysis with hydration
Adequate hydration decreases/dilutes the effect of the toxin.

Treat ATN and AIN by avoidance or removal of the nephrotoxic agent
Contrast-induced renal failure is usually transient. Attempt to avoid this problem by
hydrating pt with half normal saline 12 hrs before and after the procedure.

For postrenal failure, place a Foley then identify and remove obstruction

Refer for emergent dialysis if indicated for severe refractory
- Acidosis   - Volume Overload   - Uremia   - HyperKalemia

S **Does the pt have any personal or family history of kidney disease?**
- Diabetes mellitus (DM)
- Systemic lupus erythematosus (SLE)
- Polycystic kidney disease
- Obstructive uropathy
- Focal segmental glomerulosclerosis
- IgA nephropathy
- Hypertension (HTN)
- Glomerulonephritis (GN)
- Alport's syndrome
- Interstitial nephritis
- Postinfectious glomerulonephritis

Does the pt have any symptoms of uremia?
- Pruritus   - Anorexia   - Nausea
- Vomiting   - Singultus   - Nocturia
- Impotence   - Tremor   - Leg cramps

Does the pt have any history of volume loss?
Volume depletion from the GI tract or the kidneys can cause acute renal failure.

O **Review VS**
Look for high blood pressure.
Check orthostatics.
Tachycardia and hypotension suggest volume depletion.

Perform PE
Gen: sallow complexion
Skin: ecchymosis, epistaxis (resulting from uremic toxins causing platelet dysfunction)
Neuro: stupor, asterixis, myoclonus
Eyes: fundoscopic exam; pale conjunctiva suggests anemia
Cardio: Rubs (pericarditis), murmur, S_3, S_4 suggest fluid overload.
Pulm: Crackles, decreased breath sounds suggest fluid overload.
Abd: Palpate for enlarged kidneys.
Ext: edema

Check BUN and creatinine
To confirm the diagnosis and compare with previous values if available. This is one of the best ways to differentiate chronic from acute renal failure.

Check Mg^{2+} and phosphorus
These are often high in renal failure because of decreased excretion.

Check Ca^{2+}
Usually low because of decreased GI absorption, resistance to parathyroid hormone, and decreased $1,25 (OH)_2D_3$, which is produced by the kidneys.

Check CBC
CBC shows normocytic anemia caused by decreased erythropoietin.

Estimate glomerular filtration rate (GFR) with 24-hr urine creatinine and creatinine clearance (renal function)

$$\text{Cr Cl (mL/min)} = \frac{\text{Urine Cr (mg/dL)} \times \text{Urine vol. (mL/min)}}{\text{Plasma Cr (mg/dL)}}$$

Normal range of creatinine clearance: 95 to 105 mL/min

Obtain a renal ultrasound
Size usually < 10 cm in chronic renal failure (CRF).
Diabetes, amyloidosis, and multiple myeloma produce normal to large kidney size.

Review urinalysis
Typical specific gravity is 1.010, and blood and protein are common in CRF.
Waxy casts indicate chronic renal disease.

Check ECG
To evaluate possible pericarditis or changes caused by hyperkalemia

Chronic Renal Failure
A worsening of renal function to a GFR < 60 mL/min for longer than 3 months.

Etiologies
- DM   - HTN   - Chronic GN
- Cystic kidney disease   - Interstitial nephritis   - SLE
- HIV   - Obstructive uropathy

Treat reversible causes of chronic renal insufficiency
- Infection   - Obstruction   - Volume depletion
- Hypertension   - Congestive heart failure

Monitor I/Os
Many pts will not be oliguric until later in the disease, but it is important to monitor this and start dialysis in a timely fashion.

Prevent hyperkalemia by avoiding foods high in potassium and taking kayexalate when necessary
The kidneys normally excrete excess potassium, but in renal failure they are less effective. As a result, intake of potassium needs to be reduced.

Avoid and treat hyperphosphatemia to prevent renal osteodystrophy
Use calcium carbonate 648 mg po tid with meals when PO^{3-} is less than 6.
Use amphojel if PO^{3-} is more than 6.
Restrict foods high in phosphorus such as eggs, dairy products, and meats.
Restrict foods high in potassium such as pinto beans, bananas, tomatoes, and orange juice.

Control HTN and DM to slow progression of renal failure
Tight glycemic control
Recommend using an ACE inhibitor for DM. Avoid ACE inhibitor when Cr > 2.0.
Avoid nephrotoxins and IV contrast if possible.
Dialysis after radiocontrast dye does not prevent renal damage.

Restrict sodium intake and maintain adequate nutrition
Treat hyperlipidemia
Cardiovascular disease is the most common cause of death in pts with CRF.

Treat anemia with erythropoietin injections (Epogen) 10,000 U SQ 3 times per wk
Refer for emergent dialysis for severe refractory
- Hyperkalemia   - Acidosis   - Volume overload
Uremia (encephalopathy, pericarditis, or platelet dysfunction)

Prevent and treat uremic bleeding
DDAVP (desmopressin)—causes release of factor VIII
- Cryoprecipitate   - Conjugated estrogens

Treat uremic pruritus with antihistamines
Refer early to a nephrologist for evaluation of dialysis

S What is the clinical presentation?
Edema
+ Renal failure
These pts are hypercoagulable because of excretion of anticoagulants into the urine.
- Pulmonary embolism   - Renal vein thrombosis

Does pt have any conditions that cause membranous glomerulonephropathy?
- Diabetes   - Hepatitis B   - Hepatitis C
- Syphillis   - Amyloidosis   - Systemic lupus erythematosus (SLE)
- History of cancer: lung, breast, leukemia, lymphoma

Is the pt on any medications that can cause proteinuria?
- Captopril   - NSAIDs   - Probenacid
- D-penicillamine   - Heroin   - Gold

O Review VS
Look for hypertension as a sign of possible renal involvement (consider
  glomerulonephritis in the differential diagnosis).
Look for hypotension as a sign of decreased intravascular volume.

Perform PE
Gen: lymphadenopathy, malar rash (SLE), pale
HEENT: periorbital edema, doughy earlobes
Pulm: decreased breath sounds, crackles (Point to fluid overload and pleural effusion.)
Back: Check for flank or back tenderness. (This may suggest renal vein thrombosis and
  occurs more with membranous glomerulonephropathy.)
Abd: ascites
Ext: pitting edema

Repeat U/A to confirm proteinuria on the dipstick
Proteinuria can be present during high fevers or following vigorous activities.
Protein > 300 mg/dL and oval fat bodies are pathognomonic for nephrotic syndrome.

Check a 24-hr urine protein
The pt is instructed to void and discard the first morning urine specimen.
Then begin collecting urine up to and including the next morning's first void.
24-hr urine creatinine is used to ensure a proper collection and to calculate the
  glomerular filtration rate.
- In females, the creatinine should be from 10–15 mg/kg.
- In males, 15–20 mg/kg.

Check BUN and creatinine to look for renal insufficiency
Check serum glucose
In adults, nephrotic syndrome is highly associated with diabetes.
- Large proteinuria is often the predecessor of end-stage renal disease in these pts.

Order a lipid panel
To look for hyperlipidemia

Check serum albumin
To look for hypoalbuminemia

Order tests based on clinical suspicion
- RPR   - Hepatitis B/C
- ANA   - dsDNA

Consider imaging and workup if suspect sequelae of hypercoagulability such as deep vein thrombosis, pulmonary embolism, and renal vein thrombosis

Nephrotic syndrome is a hypercoagulable state caused by urinary loss of protein C, S, and antithrombin III.

Nephrotic Syndrome

A clinical entity, of increased permeability of the capillary basement membranes of the glomeruli, characterized by:

- Proteinuria (> 3.5 g/1.73 m^3/24 hrs)   - Hypoalbuminemia and
- Hypercholesterolemia   albuminuria
- Edema

Etiology

Membranous glomerulonephritis (most common in adults):
- Idiopathic
- Secondary:
  - Hepatitis B   - Syphilis   - Lymphoma
  - Leukemia   - Lung CA   - Breast CA

IgA nephropathy (10% present with nephrotic syndrome)

Minimal change disease (more common in children)

Membranoproliferative glomerulonephritis

Focal segmental glomerulosclerosis:
  - Heroin abusers   - HIV
  - Reflux uropahty   - Morbidly obese

SLE

Diabetes mellitus

Differential diagnosis

  - Congestive heart failure   - Cirrhosis   - Renal failure
  - Severe malnutrition   - Vasculitis   - HIV

P **Reduce edema with gentle diuresis and salt restriction**

Also carefully monitor for signs of intravascular hypovolemia, hypotension.

Reduce proteinuria with ACE inhibitors if creatinine permits

If they have Cr > 2.0, do not use ACE inhibitor (high risk of hyperkalemia in renal failure).

Treat hyperlipidemia with lipid-lowering agents to reduce the risk of cardiovascular disease

Consult Nephrology for renal biopsy and further workup

Biopsy is done when the etiology is unclear.

The treatment of nephrotic syndrome depends on the underlying cause

Primary membranous glomerulonephropathy with prednisone and cyclophosphamide

Focal segemental glomerulosclerosis with prednisone

Hepatitis B with interferon

Syphilis with penicillin

Lupus with steroids

If renal vein thrombosis is suspected, duplex ultrasound of the kidneys should be ordered. Once confirmed, pt is to be hospitalized and started on heparin

S **Is the hematuria at the beginning, end, or throughout urination?**
Hematuria seen at the beginning of urination indicates urethral bleeding.
Terminal hematuria indicates a bladder neck or prostate problem.
Hematuria throughout urination indicates an upper urinary tract problem.

What are the associated symptoms?
Dysuria, frequency, and urgency suggest cystitis.
Flank pain radiating to the groin indicates a kidney stone (rarely painless).
Symptoms such as fever and weight loss may suggest renal cell CA or vasculitis.

Is the pt menstruating?
Menstruation is a common cause of apparent hematuria in women.

Does the pt have a Foley catheter?
Placement of the catheter causes trauma to the lower GU tract.

Is there a family history of kidney disease?
Family history of polycystic kidney disease, Alport syndrome, SLE, sickle cell
History of hemoptysis associated with vasulitis (Wegener's)
Recent upper respiratory tract infection suggests IgA nephropathy.

Did the pt recently have a sore throat?
Poststreptococcal GN can occur about 10 to 21 days after a strep throat infection.
IgA nephropathy causes hematuria a week after a viral infection or with exercise.

What medicine is the pt taking?
NSAIDs and aspirin can increase the risk of bleeding.
Cyclophosphamide causes hemorrhagic cystitis.
Rifampin changes the color of the urine.

O **Review VS**
High blood pressure suggests GN.
Fever suggests infection or malignancy.

Perform a PE
Skin: Malar rash, joint pain suggest SLE; purpura, petechia suggest a vasculitis.
Cardio: Atrial fibrillation can cause arterial renal embolism.
Abd: Palpate for any masses, organomegaly.
Back: Check costovertebral angle tenderness (pyelonephritis).
Genitourinary: Check for any trauma, and perform a prostate exam in males.

Check BUN and creatinine to assess renal function
Obtain a 24-hr urine with protein and creatinine
Proteinuria is common with glomerular hematuria caused by leakage through broken
   glomerular capillaries.

Check PT and PTT to rule out any coagulopathy
Order a CBC looking for anemia, platelet count, sickle cells
Check electrolytes including calcium, phosphorus, magnesium
Look for any abnormalities such as hypercalcemia suggesting renal stones.

Review urinalysis
Dysmorphic RBCs or RBC casts suggest glomerular disease.
Crystals indicate a renal stone.
Normal sized/shaped RBCs are a sign of urinary tract bleeding.
A blood clot indicates lower tract disease in general.
Large blood on the dipstick with few RBCs suggests rhabdomyolysis.

Hematuria and pyuria without organisms suggest STD.
Hansel's stain for eosinophils in the urine to rule out acute interstitial nephritis

Check urine culture and sensitivity
If suspect infection

Check renal ultrasound to assess renal size and shape
Look for stone, hydronephrosis, or multiple cysts.

Check C4 and C3 complement level
Low complement levels are in a few diseases.

- SLE	- Membranoproliferative	- Cryoglobulinemia
- Shunt nephritis	- Poststreptococcal GN	- Subacute bacterial endocarditis

Order antistreptolysin O or anti-DNAse if poststreptococcal GN is suspected

Hematuria
Urine containing blood (RBCs)

Etiologies
Upper urinary tract (dysmorphic RBCs present):
- Glomerulonephritis from various causes:
  - Poststreptococcal glomerulonephritis
  - IgA nephropathy
  - Membranoproliferative glomerulonephritis
  - Rapidly progressive glomerulonephritides
  - Vasculitis: polyarteritis nodosa, microscopic polyangiitis, Wegener's granulomatosis, Henoch-Schönlein purpura
- Renal cell carcinoma

Lower urinary tract:
- Renal stones   - Bladder infection
- Bladder cancer   - Local trauma of urethra or lower

Other causes of red/orange urine
- Rifampin   - Oxacillin   - Myoglobinuria

If infection is present, treat and then repeat U/A
Blood may be present during a urinary tract infection and may clear after treatment.

Consider c-ANCA if Wegener's disease is suspected
Consider cryoglobulin when hepatitis C is positive
Consider antiglomerular basement membrane antibody when Goodpasture's syndrome is suspected
Order intravenous pyelogram (IVP) if the above tests are negative
IVP shows the anatomy of both the upper and lower urinary tract.

Obtain abdominal CT if mass is present on ultrasound
Spiral CT of the kidneys and ureters is a good way to identify the pathology.

Send urine cytology and order cystoscopy in pts > 40 y/o with a negative urine culture, to look for bladder cancer
Risk factors for bladder cancer include:
- Cigarette smoking   - Cyclophosphamide   - Pelvic irradiation

Finally, if you suspect glomerular disease, consider renal biopsy
If all of the above tests are negative, consider an angiogram to rule out arteriovenous malformation

S **Does the pt have any history of volume depletion?**
Vomiting and diarrhea cause volume depletion (a decrease in intravascular volume) as well as sodium depletion.
Overuse of diuretics such as furosemide or hydrochlorothiazide

Is the pt on any medications that increase the release of antidiuretic hormone (ADH)?
Antipsychotic agents, narcotics, tricyclic antidepressants

Is the pt taking any medications that can enhance the action of ADH?
- NSAIDs   - Chlorpropamide

Is the pt using any of the vasopression analogs?
- DDAVP   - Oxytocin

Has the pt recently had surgery?
Most of the time pts are on NS, usually in pain, and on narcotics, all of which can stimulate the release of ADH.

Does the pt have any history of congestive heart failure, nephrotic syndrome, or cirrhosis?
These pts retain more water than sodium.
Ask about history of:
- Myocardial infarction   - Hepatitis   - Alcoholism
- Bilateral LE edema   - RUQ pain   - ↑Abdominal girth

Does the pt have symptoms of adrenal insufficiency or hypothyroidism?
These two endocrine conditions can cause hyponatremia.

Is the pt at risk for syndrome of inappropriate ADH (SIADH)?
Pulmonary processes: cancer, pneumonia
Central nervous system processes: meningitis, tumor, head trauma

O **Check volume status looking for signs of hypovolemia**
- Hypotension   - Tachycardia   - Orthostasis
- Flat neck veins   - Poor skin turgor   - Dry mucous membrane

Look for signs of hypervolemia
- Jugular venous distention   - Hepatojugular reflex   - Ascites
- Bilateral lower extremity   - Scrotal edema
  pitting edema

Look for any evidence of cirrhosis
- Spider angiomata   - Gynecomastia   - Palmar erythema
- Parotid enlargement (alcohol abuse)

Check serum Na^+. If it is < 135 mEq/L, check urine osmolality and electrolytes
Low urine sodium (< 10 mEq/L) indicates a nonrenal cause of volume depletion.
High urine sodium (> 20 mEq/L) suggests renal solute loss.
Urine osmolality in SIADH is > 100 mOsm/kg H_2O.

Check serum glucose
This effectively rules out pseudohyponatremia from hyperglycemia:

$$Na^+_{Corrected} = Na^+_{Serum} + 1.6[(Glucose - 100)/100]$$

Check BUN and creatinine to assess renal function
An elevated BUN correlates with decreased extracellular fluid.

Check serum osmolality
If osmolality is normal, it is pseudohyponatremia caused by:
- Hyperlipidemia (triglyceride > 1000)
- Hyperproteinemia (protein > 10)
- Hyperglycemia (see formula above)

Calculate sodium deficit
Na deficit = 0.6 × total body weight × (current serum Na^+ – normal Na^+)

Check TSH and serum cortisol to rule out hypothyroidism and hypoaldosteronism
SIADH is a diagnosis of exclusion.

Hypo-osmolar Hyponatremia
Low serum sodium in the absence of confoundingly high osmotic agents such as triglycerides, proteins, or glucose.

Normo-/hyperosmolar hyponatremia represents a condition like hyperglycemia where total body sodium is unchanged, it is only redistributed or diluted.

Remember that extracellular volume is determined by total body sodium, and sodium concentration is determined by total body water.
- Therefore, changes in ECV indicate changes in total body sodium.
- And changes in serum Na^+ concentration indicate changes in total body water.

Etiologies
Hypovolemia:
- Vomiting	- Diarrhea	- Adrenal insufficiency
- Diuretics	- Salt wasting	

Euvolemia:
- SIADH	- Water intoxication

Hypervolemia:
- Renal failure	- Nephrotic syndrome
- Cirrhosis	- Congestive heart failure

If hypovolemic hyponatremia, replace fluids with normal saline
If diuresis is the cause, discontinue it and replace volume.

If hypervolemic hyponatremia, restrict Na^+ and water intake
Add diuretics to increase sodium excretion if needed.

If euvolemic hyponatremia, restrict fluid to 800 to 1000 mL of intake per day
Remember to stop all medications that can cause hyponatremia.

If the pt has hyponatremia with symptoms such as headache, disorientation, confusion, or seizure, treat with 3% NS until symptoms resolve
Symptomatic hyponatremia is an emergency, but never increase at a rate more than 1 mEq/hr to avoid central pontine myelinolysis:
- Flaccid paralysis	- Dysarthria	- Dysphagia

Acutely the goal is to reverse symptoms, not to normalize sodium.

If the pt is asymptomatic, correct slowly with fluid restriction
If fluid restriction does not work, use normal saline, lithium, or demeclocycline.

S **Does the pt have any history of volume loss?**
- Diarrhea   - Nasogastric suctioning   - Fever   - Excessive burns

Does the pt have access to water and a normal sense of thirst?
- Elderly, bedridden   - Stroke   - Dementia   - Delirium

Is pt on any medications that can cause hypernatremia?
- Lithium   - Demeclocycline   - Hypertonic NaCl or $NaHCO_3$

Does the pt have conditions that can cause central diabetes insipidus?
- Head trauma   - Neurosurgery   - Meningitis/Encephalitis   - Neoplasm

Does the pt have nephrogenic diabetes insipidus (DI)?
- Hypokalemia   - Hypercalcemia   - Amphotericin B

Has the pt been drinking salt water or ingesting salt tabs?
Salt poisoning leads to a hypervolemic hypernatremia. If hypervolemia is found on the exam (edema, hypertension), and the pt is not receiving IV saline, this is the only diagnosis.

O **Check BP, heart rate, orthostatics, and I/Os**
Hypotension and tachycardia indicate hypovolemia
Polyuria can be caused by DI or primary polydipsia.

Perform a PE
Neuro: focal neurologic deficit, altered mental status, coma
Skin: poor turgor
Ext: edema

If Na^+ > 145 mEq/L, check serum Ca^{2+} and K^+
Hypercalcemia and hypokalemia can cause nephrogenic DI.
Hypokalemia and hypertension are associated with hyperaldosteronism, which may cause borderline increases in serum sodium concentration.

Check urine osmolality
Urine osmolality < 200 mOsm/L indicates central DI.
Urine osmolality between 200 to 500 mOsm/L indicates nephrogenic DI.

Check urine sodium
Random urine sodium can help in assessing the extracellular volume (ECV). Urine Na^+ < 10 mEq/L suggests a low extracellular volume.

Consider administering a water deprivation test if you suspect DI
Give 10 μg intranasal DDAVP after water restriction to differentiate central (urine osmolality increases by at least 50%) from nephrogenic DI (no change).
Administer this test under close supervision because fluid loss can be excessive.

A **Hypernatremia**

Increased serum sodium

Remember that ECV is determined by total body sodium, and sodium concentration is determined by total body water.

- Therefore, changes in ECV indicate changes in total body sodium.
- And changes in serum Na^+ concentration indicate changes in total body water.

Etiologies

Low ECV: water loss in excess of Na^+ loss

              - Diarrhea   - Vomiting   - Sweat   - GI secretions

Normal ECV: loss of free water with no change in Na^+

- Diabetes insipidus: central or nephrogenic

High ECV: Na^+ gain in excess of water gain

- Normally iatrogenic from hypertonic saline infusion

P **If hypovolemic hypernatremia, correct hypovolemia with normal saline (NS)**

Give 500 mL to 1 L NS bolus and recheck. Repeat until hypovolemia resolves

After initial boluses have been given, calculate free water deficit.

$$\text{Water deficit:} \quad \frac{(\text{Plasma Na}^+ - \text{Desired Na}^+)}{\text{Desired Na}^+} \times 0.6 \times \text{ body weight in kg}$$

Replace with hypotonic solution (e.g., 1/2 NS or NS)

Also take into account ongoing losses of water (e.g., fever, diarrhea, diaphoresis, urine output) when calculating water deficit.

For example: You have a 70-kg male with a serum Na^+ of 165 mEq/L. You want to calculate the water deficit with a desired corrected Na^+ to be 155 mEq/L in the next 10 hrs.

- Water deficit = $(165 - 155)/155 \times 0.6 \times 70 = 2.7$ L
- Now, take into account insensible loss (from $0.5 - 1$ L/24 hrs).

Rate of correction depends on symptoms and the acuity of hypernatremia.

- If hypernatremia has been present for weeks, correct slower than in a case where the hypernatremia occurred in hrs.
- Usually give half of the volume in the first 8 hrs and then half over the next 16 hrs.
- If rate of correction is too fast, it can cause cerebral edema.

If the pt has isovolemic hypernatremia, evaluate central versus nephrogenic DI

See above.

Treat central DI with intranasal DDAVP

Be sure to replace free water.

Treat nephrogenic DI by removing the offending toxin or medication

Treat with low-sodium diet, thiazide diuretic, and replace free water.

If the pt has hypertonic hypernatremia, identify cause such as hypertonic saline and discontinue it

It is sometimes necessary to use diuretics to excrete excess Na^+, in which case water loss during such therapy needs to be replaced.

S **Does the pt have a history of GI potassium loss?**
   - Diarrhea   - Vomiting   - Laxatives   - Gastric suctioning

Is the pt taking any medicines that can cause renal potassium loss?
   - Hydrochlorothiazide   - Lasix   - Aminoglycosides
   - Amphotericin B   - Cisplatin   - Penicillins

Does the pt have any risk factors for transcellular shift of potassium?
   - Insulin   - Alkalosis   - Refeeding
   - β-adrenergic drugs such as albuterol, epinephrine
   - Hypokalemic periodic paralysis with thyrotoxicosis

Is the pt losing the potassium from the kidneys?
   - Type I renal tubular acidosis   - Diabetic ketoacidosis
   - Recovery phase of acute renal failure   - Postobstructive diuresis
   - Barter's syndrome   - Osmotic diuresis

Could this pt have hyperaldosteronism?
Consider this diagnosis in pts with hypertension, hypernatremia, and hypokalemia.
Hypokalemia without any provocation suggests hyperaldosteronism. Remember that
   aldosterone causes potassium secretion at the distal renal tubules.

Is the pt at risk for magnesium loss?
Hypomagnesemia causes hypokalemia. Treatment of hypokalemia without
   replacement of magnesium can never be achieved. Besides GI losses, renal losses can
   result from diuretics, cisplatin, and aminoglycosides.

O **Review VS and perform a PE**
Check for flaccid paralysis and hyporeflexia (can occur with potassium < 2.5).
Check for asterixis because hypokalemia can precipitate hepatic encephalopathy.
Abd exam: May have decreased or absent bowel sounds secondary to functional ileus.

Look for ECG changes
   - Flattened T-waves   - Prominent U-waves
   - ST-segment depression   - Prolonged QT

Repeat the potassium to verify the abnormality
Check BMP, Mg^{2+}, Ca^{2+}, and phosphorus
Prolonged hypomagnesemia can cause hypocalcemia from decreased parathyroid
   hormone (PTH) secretion, as well as PTH resistance.
Low Mg^{2+} decreases K^+ reabsorption across renal tubules.

Check a CBC
An elevated WBC can cause pseudohypokalemia.

Check urine potassium
To differentiate renal (> 40 mEq/24 hr) versus GI potassium (< 20 mEq/24 hr) losses

Consider further workup
If you suspect hyperaldosteronism, draw plasma renin (low) and aldosterone levels.
If there is evidence of acidosis (a low bicarbonate), think type I renal tubular acidosis
   (RTA).
Urine Cl^- < 15 mEq/L indicates GI losses (nasogastric tube suctioning, vomiting).
Urine Cl^- > 25 mEq/L suggests renal losses.

A
Hypokalemia
Low serum potassium

Etiologies
GI loss:
- Diarrhea   - Vomiting
- Laxatives   - Gastric suctioning
Renal loss:
- Type I RTA
- Diabetic ketoacidosis
- Recovery phase of acute renal failure
- Postobstructive diuresis
- Barter's syndrome
- Osmotic diuresis
- Medicines that can cause renal potassium loss:
  - Thiazide diuretics   - Furosemide
  - Aminoglycosides   - Amphotericin B
  - Cisplatin   - Penicillins
Transcellular shift of potassium
- Insulin   - Alkalosis   - Refeeding
β-adrenergic drugs: albuterol, epinephrine
Hypokalemic periodic paralysis with thyrotoxicosis

P
Eliminate and treat conditions that can cause transcellular shifts of potassium
Replace potassium.
- Oral replacement is preferred and is much safer than the IV route.
- In symptomatic, severe hypokalemia, IV KCl (10 mEq/L/hr).

Treat low Mg^{2+} with $MgSO_4$ IV or MgO po depending on severity
It is nearly impossible to replace the K^+ if the Mg^{2+} is not replaced.

In addition to replacing potassium, the underlying cause of hypokalemia should be addressed and corrected as follows
Control diarrhea, vomiting.
Discontinue diuretics.
Use a standing dose of potassium in pts on cisplatin, aminoglycosides.

Treat chronic hypokalemia (like Barter syndrome) with KCl supplement or potassium-sparing diuretics: spironolactone, triamterene, or amiloride
If hypokalemia is caused by hyperaldosteronism, a CT scan of the abdomen should be ordered to evaluate for adrenal mass
Treat hyperaldosteronism with spironolactone.
Consider consulting Endocrinology.

S **Does the pt have a personal or family history of kidney disease?**
Renal insufficiency decreases the excretion of K^+ (potassium).

Briefly review the pt's diet
Some salt substitutes (KCl) are high in potassium.
Foods that contain K^+ include pinto beans, bananas, tomatoes, and oranges.

Is the pt taking any medications that can cause hyperkalemia?
Spironolactone is a competitive inhibitor of aldosterone, which causes an increase in
   absorption of sodium and an increase in secretion of potassium.
ACE inhibitors also decrease renal excretion of potassium.
NSAIDs inhibit production of renin and aldosterone synthesis.

Does the patient use albuterol?
β-agonists such as albuterol can cause potassium to shift out of the cells.

Does the pt have any conditions that could cause hyperkalemia?
Rhabdomyolysis: trauma, statins, cocaine, alcohol
Volume contraction: With rehydration, K^+ will drop to normal or even low levels.
      - DKA   - Sepsis   - Severe dehydration

Does the pt have a history of malignancy?
Can cause tumor lysis syndrome with death and leakage of internal contents of rapidly
   overturning cancer cells into the blood stream.

Is the pt diabetic?
Diabetes mellitus can cause type IV RTA because of the defect of H+-ATPase pump in
   the collecting tubules.
Other causes of type IV RTA include obstructive uropathy and interstitial nephritis.

Is the pt fasting?
In pts who are dependent on dialysis, prolonged fasting decreases insulin secretion,
   which promotes potassium shift from intracellular to extracellular space.
In a normal individual, this amount of potassium is excreted. In a pt dependent on
   dialysis, the potassium cannot be excreted, potentially causing life-threatening
   arrhythmia.

Was it a difficult blood draw?
Hemolyzed blood specimen can cause falsely elevated K^+.
This is a diagnosis you should confirm with a repeat test showing a normal K^+.

O **Review VS and perform a general PE**
Look for evidence of muscle weakness, paralysis, or arrhythmia.

Order an ECG
ECG shows peaked T-waves, flattening or absence of P-waves, widened QRS, and
   prolonged PR interval.
   • This results in an ECG with the appearance of a sine wave.
Do not rely on ECG findings.
As the K^+ increases, the T-waves increase and then begin to decrease again.
So although the absence of peaked T-waves does not exclude significant hyperkalemia,
   their presence is nearly diagnostic.
Arrhythmia includes ventricular fibrillation and asystole.

Repeat potassium to verify result or see effect of acute treatment
Traumatic venipuncture can cause hemolysis. Look for a comment of hemolysis.

Check BUN and creatinine to assess renal function
Decreased renal function increases the risk of hyperkalemia caused by poor excretion.

Check Ca^{2+} level
It is often low in renal failure but high in conditions such as multiple myeloma.

Check CBC for anemia, leukocytosis, and thrombocytosis
Both leukocytosis and thrombocytosis can cause pseudohyperkalemia from leakage of K+ from these cells.

Check U/A
Rhabdomyolysis: Myoglobin tests as large blood in the dipstick without any RBCs on microscopy.

Check urine potassium
Hyperkalemia with urine K^+ > 30 mEq/L suggests transcellular shifts.
Hyperkalemia with urine K^+ < 30 mEq/L indicates impaired excretion.

Consider ordering a blood gas
This is a fast way to check serum potassium. Stat chemistry may take up to 1 hr to come back. Blood gas chemistry often comes back in 5 minutes.

Hyperkalemia
High serum potassium

Etiologies
Decreased cellular potassium uptake
Increased cellular potassium release

- Insulin deficiency	- Rhabdomyolysis	- Tumor lysis
- Aldosterone deficiency	- Hyperosmolality	syndrome
- β-adrenergic blockers	- Volume contraction	

Decreased renal clearance
- Acute or chronic renal failure

Differential diagnosis
Hemolyzed blood specimen: Lysis of RBCs releases the internal contents of the cells, which are high in potassium.

Quantify serum potassium level and check an ECG for changes
If there are ECG changes, give 10 mL of IV calcium gluconate over 1 minute
Stabilizes the myocardium (does not affect the potassium level)
Works in < 5 min and lasts for 30 to 60 min. Repeat prn q 3 to 5 min.

If K^+ > 7, place a cardiac monitor and give meds to move K^+ intracellularly
10 U insulin IV with an amp of D50W (monitor serum K^+ and glucose)
$NaHCO_3$ 2 mEq/kg IV over 5 to 10 min (monitor K^+)

If K^+ > 6, place cardiac monitor and give meds to increase K^+ excretion
Give kayexalate with sorbitol to enhance clearance through the GI tract.
Use IV diuretics like furosemide.

If K^+ does not improve with above management, consult renal for dialysis
Avoid meds that can cause hyperkalemia, such as NSAIDs and ACE inhibitors
Avoid foods that contain high K^+, including pinto beans, bananas, tomatoes, and orange juice

S **Does the pt have any symptoms of a lower urinary tract infection (UTI)?**
- Urgency   - Frequency   - Dysuria   - Suprapubic pain

Does the pt have any evidence of an upper UTI?
Pyelonephritis: flank pain, fever/chills, nausea/vomiting

Does the pt have any risk factors for UTI?
- Recent sexual intercourse   - Diabetes   - Pregnancy
- Foley catheter   - Anal sex   - Anatomic abnormality

O **Check VS and orthostatics**
Look carefully for any evidence of urosepsis:
- Hypotension   - Tachycardia   - Fever

Perform a general PE
Abd exam: suprapubic tenderness
Back: Check costovertebral angle for tenderness (suggests pyelonephritis).

Check a urinalysis
Positive leukocyte esterase suggests infection.
Positive nitrite also suggests infection, but some bacteria do not produce nitrate.
WBC > 5 = pyuria
RBCs are often but not always present in UTI.

Order a urine Gram stain and culture and sensitivity
E. coli is one of the most common causes of UTIs.
Look for 10^2 colonies in symptomatic females or 10^3 in symptomatic males.
Other common organisms are the following:
- Klebsiella   - Proteus   - Enterobacter
- Pseudomonas   - Serratia   - Citrobacter
Staphylococcus aureus is a rare cause of UTI and if isolated from the urine, it is normally a result of hematogenous spread.
Isolating *Streptococcus bovis* from the urine is an indication that the pt may have a colonic malignancy.

If there is fever, tachycardia, hypotension, flank pain, vomiting, or other signs of systemic or upper UTI, consider blood cultures
Try to obtain these before administering antibiotic

Check the CBC
Look for leukocytosis and bandemia, both of which suggest a systemic infection.

A **Urinary Tract Infection**
Usually bacterial (but other infectious agents like fungal and viral also occur) of the upper (kidneys) or lower (bladder) urinary system

Differential diagnosis
Lower UTI:
- Prostatitis   - Epididymitis   - Interstitial cystitis   - Urethritis
Upper UTI:
- Appendicitis   - Meningitis   - Pneumonia
- Endocarditis   - Renal stone   - Sepsis

P **If it is an uncomplicated lower UTI, treat with a three-day course of TMP/SMX**

In pregnant women, avoid TMP/SMX (in third trimester) and quinolones. Suggest a 7-day course of nitrofurantoin or first-generation cephalosporin.

For a woman with recurrent simple UTIs, prophylatic measures should be considered:
- Postcoital antibiotic; Bactrim, one single-strength tablet
- Pt self-administered treatment
- Continuous low-dose antibiotic
- Void after intercourse.
- Drink cranberry juice.
- Avoid use of diaphragm with spermicide.

Do not treat asymptomatic bacteriuria except in pts with diabetes mellitus or pregnancy.

If there is evidence that the pt has pyelonephritis, treat with 7 days of a quinolone, or 14 days with TMP/SMX, or amoxicillin-clavulanate Admit and treat for 1 to 2 days with IV antibiotics if pt has nausea, vomiting, and is unable to keep any liquid down

If the pt is not tolerating oral fluids, then he or she may not survive at home. Once pt is afebrile, switch to oral antibiotic.

If pt continues to have fever after 48 hrs of starting IV antibiotics, consider CT abdomen to rule out renal abscess

Also consider emphysematous pyelonephritis, a rare, but fatal disease if not detected early, especially in poorly controlled diabetics. It is caused by a gas-producing organism, usually *E. coli*. A KUB is usually diagnostic. Its management is antibiotics and nephrectomy.

If pt is a male with a UTI, treat with 7 days of antibiotics and perform a urologic workup if no risk factors are present (e.g., unprotected anal intercourse)

UTIs are distinctly rare in men, so when they occur, the cause needs to be investigated.
- Most commonly, prostate enlargement will be the cause.

If *Candida* is cultured from the urine in a pt with a Foley catheter, remove the Foley

If funguria persists, fluconazole 100 to 400 mg/day for 7 days is recommended. Alternatively, one can order amphotericin B bladder wash (50 mg/L continuously for 5 days.

If there is pyuria without bacteruria or hematuria, culture for *Chlamydia* and gonorrhea. Also consider tuberculosis

VI

Hematology/Oncology

S **Does the pt have any symptoms of anemia?**
- Fatigue/weakness   - Dizziness   - Decrease in work capacity
- Headache   - Dyspnea   - Palpitations or anorexia

Does the pt report blood loss?
- Hematemesis   - Melena   - Hemoptysis   - Trauma
- Hematochezia   - Postop   - Hematuria   - Menorrhagia

Does the pt have unusual cravings (pica) such as starch, clay, or ice?
A common sign of underlying anemia is strange food cravings.

Does a female pt report an abnormal menstrual cycle?
Ask about last menstrual period, duration, flow, and number of pads.

Does pt have conditions associated with anemia?
HIV risk factors   Environmental exposure (lead)
Alcohol use or intravenous drug abuse   Parasitic infection (malaria)
Chronic disease (autoimmune, infection, thyroid, liver or renal)
GI surgery (iron absorbed by distal duodenum)

Is there a family history of blood disorders?
- Sickle cell   - Thalassemia   - Kidney disease   - Autoimmune disorders

Review medications (some can cause bone marrow suppression)
- Chemotherapy   - Antibiotics   - Antiseizure medications

O **Does the pt have VS associated with hemodynamic instability?**
Tachycardia, hypotension, and positive orthostatics suggest acute blood loss.

Perform a PE
Gen: Assess nutrition and fluid status, cachexia, temporal wasting, and skin turgor.
HEENT: conjunctival pallor   *Heart*: murmur
Abd: splenomegaly   *Rectal exam*: stool guiac, hemorrhoids
Skin changes: brittle nails, jaundice   Lymph nodes

Evaluate the results of a CBC with differential
Normal Hb and Hct is 13.5 and 42, respectively, for females; 15 and 45 for males.
Mean corpuscular volume (MCV) = (Hct × 10)/RBC; normal is about 90.
- If it is microcytic anemia (MCV < 80), check a microcytic (iron) panel.
- If it is macrocytic anemia (MCV > 100), check a macrocytic panel.
Mean corpuscular hemoglobin concentration (MCHC) = Hb × 100/Hct
- Hypochromic (MCHC < 30): iron deficiency, thalassemia
- Hyperchromic (MCHC > 37): spherocytosis, newborns
RDW normal range is 11.5 to 14.5. Helpful in distinguishing thalassemia and anemia of chronic disease from the following conditions with increased RDW (> 14.5):
- Iron deficiency   - Megaloblastic anemia
- Hemoglobinopathies   - Immune hemolytic anemia
Reticulocyte count to assess function of bone marrow; it comes as a percentage
- Reticulocyte count is usually given as reticulocyte percent (normal 0.5% to 1.5%)
- Calculate the reticulocyte index (RI) to interpret:
  - RI = Retic % × (pt's Hct/45) = (normal is about 1). For example, severe anemia 1 × 21/45 = 0.467 (inappropriately normal reticulocyte count). To have a normal RI with this level of anemia requires a reticulocyte percent of about 2.2 → 2.2 × 21/45 = 1 = Normal
    - High suggest increased production; low suggest decreased production.
Look at RBC morphology (sizes, shapes, and inclusions). (See Appendix A.)

Look for markers of hemolysis
- Increased lactate dehydrogenase   - Increased bilirubin   - Schistocytes

 Anemia
A low level of circulating RBCs (Hb < 12 in females or 13.5 in males). The etiologies of anemia can be summed as uncompensated blood loss, destruction, and lack of production. Time course can be chronic to acute.

Differential diagnosis/Etiology
Check MCV and decide whether it is microcytic, normocytic, or macrocytic.
- Microcytic (MCV < 80):
  - Iron metabolism: iron deficiency, chronic disease
  - Globin synthesis: thalassemia, hemoglobinopathy
- Normocytic (80–100)
  - Increased loss/destruction: posthemorrhagic, hemolytic
  - BM infiltration: malignant, myelofibrosis, storage disease
  - Decreased erythropoietin production: renal, liver, endocrine
- Macrocytic (MCV > 100): B_{12} or folate deficiency

After identifying the type of anemia, investigate the cause. It is not enough to say iron-deficiency anemia or anemia of chronic disease. In the case of iron deficiency, at least ensure that it is not caused by chronic losses from GI cancer. One way of investigating is to check iron studies if the anemia is microcytic.
- Serum Iron: Normal 70–170
  - Increased: hemolysis (thalassemia, acute leukemia), iron poisoning, transfusion, liver disease, nephritis, hemochromatosis
  - Decreased: iron deficiency, chronic blood loss, chronic disease (systemic lupus erythematosus, rheumatoid arthritis, infection), decreased iron absorption
- Total iron binding capacity (TIBC): Normal 250–450
  - Increased: iron deficiency, blood loss, pregnancy, liver disease
  - Decreased: anemia of chronic disease (infection, renal, liver), burns, malnutrition, iron overload
- Iron Saturation = (Serum Iron ×100)/TIBC → Normal 10% to 50%
  - Increased: iron therapy, thalassemia, hemochromatosis
  - Decreased: iron deficiency, cancer, chronic disease

P   **If the pt is hemodynamically unstable, admit to a monitored bed**
If there are signs of acute blood loss, the pt should be monitored closely. If the pt is bleeding and you fluid resuscitate him or her, you should see a response in the pulse and blood pressure (correction of tachycardia and hypotension).

Place two large-bore IVs, provide aggressive fluid resuscitation, type and cross, and monitor serial CBCs
Two IVs are needed to assure that IV access is not lost if one of them fails. They are large bore so that you can give IV fluid boluses quickly and so RBCs pass smoothly. After 3 boluses of IV fluids, consider transfusing blood, especially if the hematocrit is low.

If hemodynamically stable, work up the underlying cause and treat it
Transfuse only if pt is symptomatic and there is no evidence of hemolysis.

S **Does the pt have bleeding with fever or altered mental status?**
Suspicious for thrombotic thrombocytopenic purpura (TTP)/hemolytic uremic
 syndrome (HUS), which requires immediate attention

Does the pt report any mucocutaneous bleeding?
The following suggest low platelets:
           - Spontaneous gum bleeding - Epistaxis   - GI or GU bleeding
           - Menorrhagia   - Easy bruising or rash

Review medications
Many medications cause decreased platelets:
           - Sulfonamides   - Thiazides   - Quinine
           - Heparin   - INH

When was the pt's last alcohol use?
Alcohol causes direct toxicity to bone marrow.
Chronic abuse may cause liver disease and splenomegaly (sequestration).

Does the pt have medical problems associated with low platelets?
History of HIV: Consider autoimmune-mediated etiology.
History of chronic liver disease or hepatitis: Consider splenic sequestration.

Does the pt report recent blood transfusions or fluid replacement?
After massive transfusions or fluid resuscitation, platelet counts may be low because of
 dilution.

O **Review VS and perform a PE**
Gen: Assess level of consciousness.
Skin: petechiae, purpura, ecchymosis, rash, pallor, jaundice, lymph nodes
Heart: prosthetic valve
Abd: splenomegaly, hepatomegaly

Review the results of a CBC
Thrombocytopenia is defined as platelets < 150,000.
Multiple cell lines affected (anemia, leukopenia) suggests a problem with decreased
 production.
Consider bone marrow aspirate/biopsy: Low megakaryocytes indicates decreased
 platelet production. Increased indicates likely increased destruction.

Review peripheral smear
In a pt with disease associated with accelerated destruction, look for the following:
 • Fragmented RBCs (schistocytes) suggests TTP or MAHA.
 • Large platelets suggests idiopathic thrombocytopenic purpura (ITP).

Consider further lab tests
Consider PT, PTT, and disseminated intravascular coagulation (DIC) panel to rule out
 DIC.
Consider lactate dehydrogenase, bilirubin as markers for hemolysis.
Consider a comprehensive metabolic panel to rule out renal failure.
Consider antinuclear antibody, Coomb's test if suspect autoimmune mediated.
Consider HIV, hepatitis panel if pt has risk factors.

Consider further imaging
Spleen size is often difficult to interpret, consider abdominal ultrasound.
Consider CT head in pt with altered level of consciousness.

A **Thrombocytopenia**
Low platelets are usually defined as platelets of < 150,000.

Etiologies
Splenic sequestration
Increased destruction
- Immune causes: ITP, AIHA (Evan's syndrome), drugs, systemic lupus erythematosis (SLE), HIV
- Nonimmune causes: TTP/HUS, sepsis, DIC, prosthetic heart valve
Decreased production
- Bone marrow infiltration: lymphoma, leukemia, other malignancy, myelofibrosis
- Bone marrow toxicity: alcohol, vitamin B_{12}, folate deficiency

Differential diagnosis
- DIC	- Malignant hypertension	- Vasculitis
- Severe preeclampsia	- HUS	- Infectious colitis

P **Identify and treat hematologic emergencies immediately. Admit the pt to a monitored bed if you suspect any of the following**
- TTP   - ITP   - DIC

Consider the following pentad for diagnosing TTP. You do not need all five to make a diagnosis!
- Fever	- Altered mental status	- Thrombocytopenia
- MAHA	- Renal failure	

If high suspicion of TTP, treat with plasmapheresis, prednisone I mg/kg, but DO NOT give platelet transfusion unless life threatening
Giving platelets in TTP can make the condition worse.

If high suspicion of ITP, treat with prednisone I mg/kg; may use IVIG or WinRho (if Rh-positive) if platelets < 10,000 or < 20,000 with bleeding
Do not give prednisone in HIV or if lymphoma/leukemia possible.

If suspect DIC, identify and treat the underlying etiology
DIC can be associated with sepsis.

Consider transfusion of platelets if platelet count is < 10,000 or < 20,000 with evidence of bleeding
Implement conservative measures in hemodynamically stable pts
Implement all of the following measures to minimize the risk of bleeding:
- Bed rest, stool softener, cough suppressants, padded bed rails
- Avoid NSAIDs and aspirin.
Withdraw any medications that could potentially be causing the problem (see above).
Vitamin supplementation for pts with decreased production includes:
- Thiamine 100 mg bid, folate 1 mg qd, and multivitamins

S **Does the pt report bleeding?**

One of the most common reasons pts seek medical treatment is for spontaneous
bleeding (e.g., nose bleeds, hematemesis, melena).
This bleeding commonly represents platelet dysfunction.

Does the pt have symptoms related to hyperviscosity?

Increased blood volume and sticky cells cause stasis.

- Vertigo   - Tinnitus   - Headaches
- Visual changes   - Recurrent thrombosis

Does the pt have pruritus, especially after a warm shower?

Pruritus is a common complaint and is often caused by an increased release
of histamine.

Does the pt report skin changes?

Erythromelalgia, defined as painful burning and erythema of the hands, is common.

Does the pt have a medical history suggestive of a secondary cause?

A pt with any of the following is at risk for secondary polycythemia:

- Smoker   - Chronic lung disease   - Congenital heart disease
- Renal disease - Recent relocation to high-altitude region

Is the pt taking any medications?

Diuretics cause contraction of plasma volume and increased hematocrit.

O **Look for VS suggestive of secondary causes of polycythemia**

Obese pts with high blood pressure and large necks are at risk for obstructive sleep
apnea (OSA).
Pulse oximetry:

- < 92% suggests lung or heart disease
- Normal measurement is typical of smoker polycythemia.

Perform a PE

HEENT: funduscopic exam (engorged retinal veins)
Abd: splenomegaly

- Lack of splenomegaly suggests a secondary cause.
- *Skin*: ruddy complexion, plethora or cyanosis

Review the CBC with differential

Common abnormalities include overproduction of cell lines.

- Leukocytosis (basophilia, eosinophilia)
- RBC
  - Males: Hgb > 17; Hct > 50%
  - Females: Hgb > 15; Hct > 45%
- Thrombocytosis

What are the results of RBC mass and erythropoietin (EPO) levels?

A pt with elevated Hct should have RBC mass measured.

- Normal RBC mass: males 26–34; females 21–29
- High normal RBC mass suggests spurious polycythemia.

If RBC mass is elevated, check EPO level to differentiate between primary versus
secondary causes:

- EPO low or absent suggests polycythemia vera.
- EPO high suggests a secondary cause.

Consider checking venous blood gas
Smoking causes elevated carboxyhemoglobin.

Consider alkaline phosphatase, uric acid, and vitamin B$_{12}$
These markers are commonly elevated in polycythemia vera.

Consider a renal ultrasound or CT abdomen/pelvis
A pt suspected of an EPO-secreting mass should have further imaging to look for hepatoma or renal mass.

Consider pulmonary function test and/or sleep study
A pt with risk factors for chronic obstructive pulmonary disease (COPD) or OSA should have further diagnostic studies to rule out underlying lung disease.

Polycythemia
Increased number of RBCs in the blood

Etiologies
Polycythemia vera
Polycythemia from secondary causes
  • Smoking (normal pulse oximetry, high EPO, COHb high)
  • Hypoxia pulse oximetry < 92% suggests coronary heart disease, right-to-left shunt, chronic lung disease
  • EPO-secreting mass
Hepatoma, uterine leiomyoma, renal cyst, cerebellar angioma
Renal disease (polycystic kidney disease)

Identify pts with secondary causes of polycythemia
Treat underlying cause:
  - Smoking cessation   - Continuous positive airway pressure or
  - Home oxygen (COPD)   Bipap (OSA)
                        - Surgical resection (EPO-secreting mass)

Treat polycythemia vera with pt education and minimize risks of hyperviscosity
Phlebotomy is the treatment of choice.
  • One unit removed per wk for goal Hct < 45.
  • Low-iron diet
  • Allopurinol for hyperuricemia
  • Benadryl, H$_1$ blocker for pruritus
  • Anagrelide used for thrombocytosis

Consider using hydroxyurea (myelosuppressive agent)
If increased phlebotomy requirement, thrombocytosis, intractable pruritus.

S **Does the pt report any easy bleeding?**

Pts with congenital coagulation disorders bleed easily, especially after trauma, surgery, tooth extractions, or any invasive procedure.

Bleeding into joints and muscles is common in hemophiliacs with minor trauma.

Does the pt have a family history of bleeding disorders?

Hemophilia A and B are both X-linked disorders.

Does the pt report recent bleeding?

- Hemoptysis   - Melena   - Hematochezia
- Hematemesis   - Menorrhagia   - Hematuria
- Easy bruising   - Epistaxis   - Gum bleeding

Does the pt have joint pain?

Hemophilia pts may have hemarthrosis with pain in weight-bearing joints.

Review medications

Ask specifically about medicines such as warfarin or heparin.

Does the pt have risk factors for developing an acquired coagulopathy?

Disseminated intravascular coagulation (DIC): Fever/chills, fatigue, or weight loss suggest infection or malignancy; also consider complication of pregnancy/retained abortion.

History of liver or renal disease

Vitamin K deficiency: Assess nutritional status (anorexia, weight loss, malabsorption, homeless).

O **Does the pt have VS suggestive of infection or sepsis?**

- Fever   - Tachycardia   - Hypotension

Perform a good general PE, looking specifically for the following

Abd: splenomegaly

Joints: hemarthrosis

Skin:

- Ecchymosis
- Petechiae/purpura
- Evidence of chronic liver disease (spider angiomata, jaundice)
- Bleeding from venipuncture or catheter sites

Review the pt's CBC

Leukocytosis, especially with left shift, indicates infection.

- Blood, urine, sputum cultures, and CXR to investigate source

Thrombocytopenia (common in DIC and sepsis)

- Check fibrinogen level (low or inappropriately normal in DIC).

Pts with anemia should have a further workup. (See Anemia, p. 90.)

Evaluate the PT and PTT results

Review the coagulation cascade: PT (**W**arfarin: **E**xtrinsic) → 7\ 10—2(5)—1—Clot/ PTT (**H**eparin: **I**ntrinsic) → 12—11—9(8)

- Factor 8 is a cofactor for factor 9, and factor 5 is a cofactor for factor 2.
- The figure demonstrates that PT and PTT have factors 10, 5, 2, and 1 in common (when these factors are involved, both will be elevated).

Prolonged PT, normal PTT = Low factor 7

- Coumadin therapy   - Mild liver disease   - Early vitamin K deficiency

Prolonged PTT, normal PT = Low factor 12, 11, 9, or 8

- Heparin therapy   - Lupus anticoagulant
- Hemophilia A or B   - Von Willebrand disease

Prolonged PT and PTT = Low factor 10, 5, 2, or 1
  - DIC   - Liver or renal disease
  - Primary fibrinolysis   - Vitamin K deficiency (Vitamin K
                                          dependent factors are 2, 7, 9, 10.)

What do the liver and renal function tests reveal?
Liver and renal disease are common causes for coagulopathy resulting from decreased
  synthesis or retention of coagulation factors.

Consider Factor VIII, IX level
Males with a family history of easy bleeding should be evaluated for hemophilia.

 Coagulopathy
A condition in which an abnormality of the clotting cascade leads to an increased risk
  of bleeding and is reflected in abnormal PT and/or PTT.

Differential diagnosis
Congenital disorders
            - Factor VIII deficiency (hemophilia A)   - Factor IX deficiency
            - Von Willebrand disease   (hemophilia B)
            - Platelet dysfunction disorders
Acquired disorders
            - DIC   - Vitamin K deficiency   - Leukemia
            - Liver disease   - Coumadin or heparin therapy   - Primary fibrinolysis
            - Renal disease   - ITP   - TTP/HUS

P **If you suspect a life-threatening condition, admit the pt to a
monitored bed**
Carefully review vital signs for signs of hypovolemia.

Look at a peripheral smear for fragmented RBCs to decide whether
this is hemolysis or blood loss
Transfusion is not always the answer. In cases of hemolytic anemia, it can actually
  exacerbate the problem.

If you suspect DIC, treat the underlying cause and give necessary
supportive care
Common underlying causes are sepsis; deliver fetus.
Can give fresh frozen plasma (FFP), cryoprecipitate, and platelets in cases of
  hemorrhage.
Use IV heparin for thrombotic events.

After ruling out DIC, consider primary fibrinolysis and
uncontrolled bleeding
May use Amicar to optimize platelet action.

Avoid ASA and other antiplatelet factors
Hemophilia A involves replacement of factor VIII and ddAVP
Prophylactic infusions of factor VIII before dental procedures and joint replacements

Hemophilia B is treated with FFP
FFP contains, among other things, Factor IX.

Optimize treatment of liver or renal disease
Treat Vitamin K deficiency with 10 mg SQ

S   Is there any shortness of breath or chest pain?

The greatest complication of deep vein thrombosis (DVT) is pulmonary embolism (PE), which warrants prompt action.

Has there been any recent prolonged bed rest or immobility?
Risk factors for DVT include:
- Recent surgeries	- Myocardial infarction
(especially orthopedic)	- Air or bus travel of
- Stroke	long duration

Are there any risk factors for hypercoagulable states?
Malignancies: prostate, lung, ovary, cervical, colon, stomach, pancreas
Nephrotic syndrome
Oral contraceptives usage

Is there a known family history of DVT?
Inherited causes of hypercoagulable states include:
- *The Factor V Leiden mutation*: Factor V is normally degraded by activated protein C. This mutation is also known as activated protein C resistance (APCR), an autosomal-dominant trait carried by 5% of the population. It is most common in whites.
- *Hyperhomocysteinemia*: Mutation may lead to an excessive amount of this amino acid metabolite, leading to both arterial and venous thrombotic episodes. It occurs in approximately 5% to 7% of the population and usually presents in the third or fourth decade.
- Deficiencies of antithrombin III, protein C, and protein S do occur but are far more rare than the previous two conditions.

Are there any prior episodes of a DVT?
Include information about confirmation of diagnosis and prior treatment with anticoagulation and duration.
Recurrent DVT after proper anticoagulation mandates lifelong anticoagulation or filter placement to prevent further DVT and PE.

O   Check VS
Low blood pressure ≡ think pulmonary embolism.
- Tachypnea   - Tachycardia   - Low O_2 saturation

Check pt's leg(s) for signs of DVT. Physical findings are usually nonspecific
- Leg pain	- Tightness	- Edema
- Erythema	- Palpable cord	

- Homan's sign (pain with dorsiflexion of ankle); sensitivity is only about 50%.

Perform Duplex ultrasound of affected leg, looking for evidence of DVT
Highly specific and sensitive for DVT
Signs include lack of spontaneous flow in vein, absence of increased flow velocity with compression veins more distally, and inability to collapse vein with compression.

Check to see if one or both legs are involved
Bilateral leg involvement suggests either a cardiac (heart failure), hepatic, or renal (nephrotic syndrome) etiology rather than DVT.

A **Deep Vein Thrombosis**

Virchow's triad for risk of DVT is immobility, vascular damage, and hypercoagulability. Although it usually occurs in the legs, it should be considered in any extremity. The use of duplex ultrasound is diagnostic. History aids more in discovering the etiology. Physical exam is not always useful in these pts.

Differential diagnosis

- Lymphedema   - Myxedema   - Cellulitis
- Muscle strain   - Baker cyst rupture

P **First, decide whether to anticoagulate this pt**

Contraindications to anticoagulation include:

- Recent GI bleed
- Stroke
- Recent craniotomy

Otherwise, begin anticoagulation with heparin

Unfractionated heparin starting with an IV bolus of 100 units/kg (maximum 5000 units) and continue at a rate of 10 units/kg/hr. Check PTT after 6 hrs and adjust for a goal PTT of 1.5 to 2.0

OR

Low-molecular-weight heparin, such as enoxaparin, at 1 mg/kg SQ bid. This method is becoming more popular because of less need to monitor PTT.

Monitor platelets daily. If decreasing, consider heparin-induced thrombocytopenia.

Then, administer oral warfarin

Start with warfarin 5 mg po qd. Monitor international normalized ration (INR) and adjust for a goal rate of 2.0 to 3.0.

- Warfarin is a difficult drug to maintain in the therapeutic range because effects are not seen until 2 days after each dose, it has multiple drug interactions, and it even interacts with certain foods. Therefore, INR must be checked frequently.

Continue heparin (in either form) until warfarin reaches therapeutic levels, and then discontinue.

Arrange for outpatient appointment with an anticoagulation clinic before discharge to continue monitoring INR and adjust warfarin dose accordingly.

Continue treatment for 3 to 6 months on initial episode of DVT; if this is not the first event, administer warfarin lifelong.

If anticoagulation is contraindicated, consider vena caval filter placement to prevent a PE
Send off blood tests to assess for the genetic hypercoagulable states noted above

S **Does the pt have any "B" symptoms?**

The presence of any of the following is associated with a worse prognosis:
- Fevers known as Pel-Ebstein occur in a cyclic pattern.
- Drenching night sweats to the point of having to change the sheets
- Unintentional weight loss, 10% or more of body weight over 6 months

Does the pt report any painless lymphadenopathy?
Common in Hodgkin's lymphoma (HL) and non-Hodgkin's lymphoma (NHL).

Does the patient have any systemic symptoms?
- Malaise   - Weakness   - Marked fatigue

Does the pt report pruritus?
Common with HL (especially the nodular sclerosing) usually worse after
  bathing/showering

Does the pt report any respiratory symptoms?
A pt may present with a dry cough or shortness of breath.

Does pt have abdominal pain?
Early satiety or abdominal pain may suggest splenomegaly.

Does pt report diffuse body pain with alcohol ingestion?
Thought to be caused by eosinophil infiltration of tumor sites (HL).

Does the pt have any risk factors for HIV?
AIDS is common with B-cell lymphomas.

Does the pt have a history of a previous infection?
History of any of the following infections increases the likelihood of lymphoma:
- Epstein-Barr virus: HL and NHL (African Burkitt's)   • Hepatitis C: NHL
- Human T-lymphotropic virus: T-cell lymphomas   • *H. pylori*: gastric
                                                      lymphoma

Is there a history of autoimmune disorders?
Pts with RA, SLE, and Sjögren's syndrome are at increased risk for developing
  lymphoma.

O **Review VS and perform a PE**

Abd: splenomegaly, hepatomegaly   *Skin*: lymph nodes (size, consistency, tenderness)

Review CBC with differential
Malignancy of cell lines vary in presentation.
- Lymphopenia   - Leukocytosis   - Thrombocytosis
- Eosinophilia   - If there is bone marrow invasion, expect pancytopenia.

Look for abnormal liver and renal function tests
Abnormal values suggest organ involvement.

Check a lactate dehydrogenase (LDH) and uric acid level
LDH serves as a marker for the bulk of tumor.
High uric acid level suggests high cell turnover and risk for tumor lysis (see below).

Evaluate chemistry panel, phosphorus, and calcium
Common abnormalities with tumor lysis are high K, high P, and low Ca.

Consider CXR
Look for pleural effusions and hilar or mediastinal lymphadenopathy.

Consider CT of the chest, abdomen, and pelvis
To evaluate extent of disease

Consider excisional node biopsy
Entire node is needed to evaluate architecture and type of lymphoma.
- Fine-needle aspiration is not sufficient for diagnosis.

Consider bilateral bone marrow biopsy
To evaluate whether bone marrow is involved

Consider lumbar puncture in HIV pts or if you suspect Burkitt's
Consider MUGA scan to evaluate ejection fraction (prechemotherapy)

A **Lymphoma**
Cancer of lymphoid tissue is often divided into NHL and HL (Table 7).

P **Identify life-threatening complications**
         - Acute leukemia (see Leukemia, p. 102)   - Tumor lysis syndrome

Identify and treat tumor lysis syndrome promptly
Tumor lysis syndrome is the result of rapid death of tumor cells.
IV fluid resuscitation, allopurinol, alkalinize urine (add HCO_3 to fluids), loop diuretics as needed, management of electrolyte abnormalities

Treat NHL based on histologic grade
Low-grade NHL:
- Watch and wait or chemotherapy with or without radiation

Intermediate or high-grade NHL:
- Chemotherapy (CHOP) plus radiation or chemotherapy alone
- HLA-matched allograft bone marrow transplant

HL Stages
Stage I: single lymph node
Stage II: 2 or more lymph nodes same side diaphragm
- "B" indicates "B" symptoms.   • "A" indicates absence of "B" symptoms.

Stage III: more than 1 extranodal sites (liver, bone marrow, brain, and lung)
Stage IV: Diffuse involvement

Treat HL based on staging
Stage I and IIA: radiation alone
- With large mediastinal mass, radiation plus chemotherapy.

Stage IIB or IIIA: radiation +/− chemotherapy
Stage IIIB or IV: chemotherapy (MOPP, ABVD)
- Consider autologous bone marrow transplant.

Table 7 Types of Lymphoma	
Non-Hodgkin's Lymphoma	**Hodgkin's Lymphoma**
Low grade	Lymphocyte predominance
Small lymphocytic/CLL	Mixed cellularity
Follicular, small or mixed	Nodular sclerosing
Intermediate	Lymphocyte depleted
Follicular, large cell or small cleaved	
Diffuse, mixed or large	
High grade	
Immunoblastic or lymphoblastic	
Small noncleaved (Burkitt and non-Burkitt)	

S

Does the pt have any risk factors for leukemia?
Previous treatment for malignancy is one of the largest risk factors for leukemia.
  - Use of alkylating agents (cyclophosphamide, melphalan)
  - Irradiation
Other risk factors include radiation exposure (Hiroshima, Chernobyl) and smoking.
Down syndrome (trisomy 21), neurofibromatosis, and Fanconi syndrome also increase
  the risk.

Is the pt experiencing any systemic symptoms?
Malaise, weakness, fever, weight loss, and night sweats are common "B" symptoms.
  • Often they confer a worse prognosis.

Ask the pt about bruising, epistaxis, gum bleeding, hematochezia, or menorrhagia
As malignant cells infiltrate the bone marrow, cellular production decreases. Often
  symptoms of thrombocytopenia will be the first sign of malignancy.

Ask the pt about recurrent infections
This would be a sign of immune system impairment, also common in leukemia.

O

Review VS
Low-grade fevers are common in leukemia. In neutropenia, fever indicates infection.
Hypotension, tachycardia, and orthostatics indicate an unstable pt; transfer to the ICU.
Tachypnea and hypoxia are signs of pulmonary leukostasis.

Perform a PE
Gen: Assess level of consciousness; pts should not be altered.
HEENT: Look for conjunctival and mucosal pallor.
  • Retinal hemorrhages and gingival hyperplasia indicate AML.
Neck: Cervical lymphadenopathy may indicate chronic lymphocytic leukemia (CLL).
Lungs: Rales may indicate leukostasis or a pneumonia.
Heart: Tachycardia and a systolic ejection murmur are common in anemic pts.
Abd: Hepatosplenomegaly likely indicates myeloid leukemias either acute or chronic.
Skin: Petechiae and ecchymoses are common findings of thrombocytopenia.
Be sure to check the axillae, groin, and epitrochlear for lymphadenopathy.

Check CBC with differential with a peripheral smear
Although leukemia can be seen with any CBC, pancytopenia or anemia/
  thrombocytopenia with leukocytosis are the most common findings.
Presence of circulating blasts on the smear is virtually diagnostic of leukemia.

Check a complete chemistry panel
Serum potassium, phosphorus, lactate dehydrogenase, and uric acid may all be
  elevated, sometimes markedly, as indicators of large cell volume turnover.
As serum phosphorus increases, serum calcium tends to decrease.

Check PT/PTT, fibrinogen, and D-dimer studies
Disseminated intravascular coagulation (DIC) is common in APL.

Order a CXR
This will rule out mediastinal involvement and pulmonary leukostasis.

Perform a bone marrow biopsy
Biopsy is required for the diagnosis of leukemia. It should be hypercellular with more
  than 30% blasts. Immunohistochemical stains can be performed to complete the
  diagnosis.

A   **Leukemia (Table 8)**
Literally means "white blood," an old term given to those diseases that may increase circulating white blood cells. Can be acute or chronic and lymphocytic or myeloid. Both ITP and aplastic anemia can look like leukemia on the initial CBC.

P   **Identify and treat hematologic emergencies; admit pt to monitored bed**
Blast crisis: blood blasts > 100,000; causes leukostasis (pulmonary, cerebral, or GI).
  • Perform cranial irradiation for cerebral involvement.
  • Perform leukapheresis and start hydroxyurea and allopurinol; alkalinize the urine.
  • Avoid blood tranfusion because this may increase viscosity.
DIC (acute promyelocytic leukemia)
  • Give IV cryoprecipitate, fresh frozen plasma, and platelets to stop bleeding.
Consider Amicar, an agent that stimulates production of von Willebrand's factor.
Tumor lysis syndrome (see Lymphoma, p. 100)
For suspected sepsis, panculture the pt, start broad-spectrum antibiotics, and give pressors as needed.

Refer all pts to heme, but chemotherapy for ALL generally includes daunorubicin, prednisone, vincristine, and asparaginase
Most AML therapies include Ara-C + daunorubicin. There is one special case
APL (M3): Ara-C + trans-retinoid acid (ATRA): leads to high remission/cure rate!

For pts with CML, allogenic BMT is the only hope of cure
Hydroxyurea therapy may prevent rising white counts.
Without BMT, CML will eventually result in blast crisis and death.

In general, there is no cure for CLL. Therapy is indicated only if there is symptomatic lymphadenopathy, organ involvement, cytopenias, or systemic symptoms

Table 8 Types of Leukemia	
Lymphocytic	**Myeloid**
Acute lymphocytic leukemia (ALL)	**Acute myelogenous leukemia (AML)**
Childhood pre-B cell (L1)	Undifferentiated (M0)
Adult pre-B cell (L2)	Myeloblastic (M1)
B-cell (Burkitt's type) (L3)	Myeloblastic with differentiation (M2)
T-cell (L1, L2)	Promyelocytic (M3); t(15:17)
Chronic lymphocytic leukemia (CLL)	Myelomonocytic (M4)
B-cell	Monoblastic (M5)
T-cell	Erythroleukemia (M6)
Large granular lymphocytic	Megakaryoblastic (M7)
Hairy cell	**Chronic myelogenous leukemia (CML)**
	Almost always Philadelphia
	chromosome (t(9;22)) positive

Does the pt report changes in a breast mass?
Most breast lesions are first detected by self-examinations (> 90%).
Details of mass should include:
- When the mass was first detected
- Changes in size, consistency, tenderness, skin
- History of abnormal breast mass in past (fine-needle aspiration [FNA], biopsy, surgery)

Does the pt have risk factors for breast cancer?
Family history of breast cancer (BRCA-1 or BRCA-2), Li-Fraumeni syndrome
Female gender (150:1 F:M)
Early age of menarche, late age of first pregnancy, late age of menopause
Diet may play a role, but this is currently controversial.
Moderate alcohol intake (mechanism unclear)
Use of oral contraceptives (OCPs) or hormone replacement therapy (HRT)
Previous radiation exposure

Is the pt currently breastfeeding?
Nursing predisposes to infections that may cause breast mass.

Does the pt give a history of recent trauma to breast?
Fat necrosis is common after trauma; may present as skin changes and breast mass.

Has the pt had a breast surgery?
If so, consider complications such as scarring or rupture of implant.

Has the pt had menopause or removal of her ovaries?
If the pt has functioning ovaries, then many of the benign masses are still on the differential: fibrocystic change, fibroadenoma, and phyllodes tumor.

Does the pt have VS suggestive of infection such as fever?
A breast abscess is a common cause of breast mass.

Perform a PE
Breast (examine pt sitting and supine): skin changes (induration, dimpling, erythema), nipple discharge, palpable mass (note size, consistency, tenderness)
Lymph nodes: axillary or supraclavicular lymph nodes

Breast mass
Common finding in women of all ages. The goal of the workup is to differentiate benign breast masses from breast cancer.

Differential diagnosis of breast mass
Breast carcinoma: a very common cause of cancer in women
Fibrocystic breast disease: presents as intermittently painful mass/masses during premenstrual cycle. Usually occurs in women receiving some form of estrogen either from ovaries, OCPs, or HRT.
Fibroadenoma: 1 to 5 cm, nontender, round, rubbery, mobile, benign mass of the breast that does not change during menses, and generally resolves after menopause. As with fibrocystic disease, usually occurs in women on estrogen.
Phyllodes tumor: rapidly growing fibroadenoma-like mass that can be either benign or malignant, usually treated with local excision and no lymph node dissection in either case (malignant form metastasizes to the lungs, not the lymph nodes). Will recur if not completely excised.

Fat necrosis: a rare cause of breast mass, with dimpling or induration of overlying skin, usually caused by trauma; important because it is clinically very similar to breast carcinoma.

Breast abscess/cellulitis: an infection causing an erythematous, tender area with or without induration, underlying mass, or fluctuance. Usually caused by *Staphylococcus aureus*. More common in breastfeeding women.

Lymphadenopathy: should be worked up carefully to differentiate benign from malignant causes: infection, metastases of solid tumors, lymphoma

Complication of breast surgery: scar, keloid, ruptured breast implant

P **If a questionable mass is found, first do an ultrasound in young women or a mammogram in postmenopausal women**
An ultrasound is more effective in evaluating younger women because of the higher amount of connective tissue in their breasts.

If a questionable mass is found on imaging or exam, perform a biopsy
For cystic masses use FNA, but for more suspicious masses refer to surgery.
- Simple cyst: fluid-filled requires no further workup
- Everything else: requires FNA, core-needle, or excisional biopsy

Cystic lesion with no residual mass: examine color of fluid.
- Clear or green color, repeat breast exam in 4 to 6 weeks.
- Bloody fluid or abnormal cytology: proceed to excisional biopsy.
- Malignant cells (see Breast Cancer, p. 106)

If the mass is suggestive of fibrocystic disease, consider FNA and recommend a supportive bra and avoidance of caffeine. Consider danazol if the pain is severe
Consider biopsy if the FNA is bloody, the mass persists, or recurs.
Danazol suppresses FSH and LH and is also used in endometriosis.

If lesion is consistent with fibroadenoma, then nothing needs to be done
For an unclear diagnosis, excision is warranted.

If phyllodes tumor is diagnosed, it should be excised
If fat necrosis or breast abcess is diagnosed, biopsy should still be performed to confirm diagnosis
Treatment with antibiotics that cover *Staphylococcus aureus* (oxacillin or dicloxacillin)

Educate all pts about breast cancer and benign breast masses. Give reassurance when appropriate and explain how to perform breast exams
Explain that the breast exam should be performed once a month about 1 week after menses (when the breasts are generally less tender).
- Examine the entire breast from sternum to midaxillary line from ribs to clavicle, with special attention to not miss the "tail of the breast," the upper outer quadrant (which extends into the axilla), because this is where more than half of breast cancers occur.
- The breasts should also be examined in the mirror, looking for dimpling of overlying skin.

S

How old is the pt?
Two-thirds of pts with breast cancer are older than 50 y/o.

What were the pt's ages of menarche and menopause (if postmenopausal)?
Early menarche and late menopause are associated with an increased risk of breast cancer.

Has the pt ever had breast cancer in the past?
If there is a personal history of breast cancer, there is a risk of recurrence.

Has the pt ever had a breast biopsy before and, if so, what were the results?
A finding of atypical hyperplasia on previous biopsy is also an increased risk of cancer.

Has a first-degree relative had breast cancer and, if so, how old was she?
The presence of breast cancer in a first-degree relative increases the risk some 300% to 400%.
A diagnosis of breast cancer at a young age (< 60 years) could indicate a genetic mutation in either the BRCA-1 or BRCA-2 genes. Carriers of these genes have an extremely high risk.

Has the pt noticed a mass in either breast or puckering or dimpling of the skin?
These can be physical signs of active malignancy.

Has the pt had any nipple discharge and, if so, what kind?
Bloody nipple discharge has a high concordance with infiltrating ductal carcinoma.
Other types of nipple discharge may or may not be associated with malignancy.

O

Perform a breast exam: visualize the breasts with the arms overhead and on the hips with the shoulders forward, to examine the axillae, and then to palpate the breasts
Early findings: palpable firm irregular nodule or breast mass, or sometimes no findings at all
Late findings: axillary lymphadenopathy, edema, immobile breast mass, bone pain, skin or nipple retraction

Order a mammogram
Routine screening each year after 40 years of age, and earlier with those with higher risk factors.
Abnormal findings most often occur (60%) over the upper lateral quadrant of breast mass.

Order and follow up on ultrasound-guided needle biopsy results
Infiltrating ductal carcinomas are the most common (85%), but other possible histologic types include invasive lobular (6% to 8%) and noninvasive intraductal or lobular in situ (5%).

Consider ordering the following laboratory analyses
CBC: May present with anemia.
Liver function test: Elevation could signify hepatic metastases.
Estrogen receptor, progesterone receptor on tumor:
  • If positive: less aggressive cancer; may be more amenable to hormonal treatment
Human epidermal growth factor receptor-2 (her-2) status on the tumor
  • If positive: pt may respond to Herceptin, a monoclonal antibody therapy

Continue workup to look for metastases when clinically indicated
Chest x-ray for pulmonary metastases
CT of brain or liver if suggestion of metastases is present
Bone scan to assess for bony metastases or elevated alkaline phosphatase or calcium

Carcinoma of the breast
Be sure to classify the stage of the cancer, because this has implications on treatment and prognosis, and survival. Also, determine the type of carcinoma (e.g., ductal, lobular).

TNM Classification for breast cancer
Tumor
- T1: tumor ≤ 2 cm
- T2: tumor 2–5 cm
- T3: tumor > 5 cm
- T4: tumor of any size that extends to chest wall or skin
Lymph nodes
- N0: no lymph node metastases
- N1: axillary lymph nodes are (+) on biopsy, but mobile on palpation
- N2: axillary lymph nodes are (−) on biopsy, fixed on palpation
- N3: internal mammary lymph nodes are (+)
Metastases
- M0: no distant metastases present
- M1: (+) distant metastases present

Confirm suspected metastases with biopsy; many diseases can mimic metastatic breast on a scan
Staging of breast cancer based on TNM classification
Stage I: T1,N0,M0
Stage IIA: T0,N1,M0; T1,N1,M0; T2,N0,M0
Stage IIB: T2,N1,M0; T3,N0,M0; T2,N2,M0; T3,N1/2,M0
Stage IIIA: T0,N2,M0; T1,N2,M0
Stage IIIB: T4, any N,M0; any T,N3,M0
Stage IV: M1, any T/N

Await tumor histology for other prognostic variables
Estrogen/progesterone receptor (+) tumors: less aggressive, likely to respond to hormones
Her-2-neu receptor (+): more aggressive tumor, will likely respond to Herceptin
High-grade tumors have a poorer prognosis than low-grade tumors.
Lobular carcinoma in situ: cancer likely in the contralateral breast; do bilateral mastectomy.

Treat based on staging
For stages I, II, or III, the pt will require:
- Lumpectomy with axillary lymph node dissection and postoperative radiation
  OR
- Modified radical mastectomy with adjuvant chemotherapy and hormonal therapy such as Arimidex or tamoxifen (for hormone receptor (+) tumor)
Chemotherapy regimens vary, but they will likely include doxorubicin and paclitaxel.
Pts with stage IV disease are considered incurable. Remission may occur with palliative radiotherapy and hormonal therapy.

S Is there a history of smoking?

Carcinoma of the lung is strongly associated with smoking and can be dose-dependent.

Multiply the number of packs of cigarettes smoked per day by the number of years smoking to come up with "pack-years" of smoking, a useful way to quantify pt's smoking.

Is there any past exposure to asbestos, radon gas, arsenic, chromium, or nickel?

These are all environmental risk factors for developing lung cancer.

Is there a history of pulmonary fibrosis, sarcoidosis, or chronic obstructive pulmonary disease?

There is a higher associated risk of lung cancer with these diseases.

Does the pt have any general or specific symptoms associated with lung cancer?

In addition to weight loss and anorexia, chronic cough and hemoptysis can often be seen.

Bony pain in the chest, back, or pelvis is an ominous sign of possible metastasis.

Headaches, nausea, vomiting, altered mental status, or seizures suggest brain metastasis.

O Perform a PE

Cachexia: Muscle wasting that is most noticeable in the temporal area of the face (temporal wasting) is more likely to be seen with advanced or long-standing history of carcinoma.

Superior vena cava syndrome: Engorgement/erythema of the head and upper extremities, caused by obstruction of the superior vena cava, requires prompt attention.

Horner syndrome: The triad of ptosis, miosis, and anhidrosis of one eye stems from involvement of the inferior cervical ganglion and sympathetic chain on the ipsilateral side.

  • Lung cancer causing Horner's syndrome is often called a Pancoast tumor.

Digital clubbing can also be seen.

Pleural effusion, characterized by decreased breath sounds and dullness to percussion, can be seen in advanced lung cancer, as can findings of obstructive pneumonia.

Obtain a CXR

Lung cancer is often represented as a white mass on the x-ray.

Obtain and review chest and liver CT, PET scan, MRI of the brain, and bone scan

Elements of special note include the size of tumor, number of nodules, presence or absence of effusion, and location of affected lymphadenopathy.

Once tissue confirmation of malignancy is confirmed, PET scan can identify metabolically active sites of metastases in mediastinal nodes.

MRI of the brain and a bone scan can identify areas of distant metastases.

Obtain pathologic tissue evidence of carcinoma

Centrally located lesions can be biopsied by bronchoscopy, whereas transthoracic needle biopsy assisted by CT will be more appropriate in a more peripherally located lesion.

If a pleural effusion is present, consider thoracentesis to obtain possible malignant cells.

Carcinoma of the lung

If pathology is available, be sure to characterize the carcinoma as either small cell or non–small cell carcinoma. Small cell is associated with an aggressive course and poor prognosis.

TNM Classification for non–small cell carcinoma of lung

Tumor:
- T1: < 3cm in size
- T2: > 3 cm, or in main bronchus but > 2 cm from carina or invades visceral pleura
- T3: in chest wall, diaphragm, or pericardium or in main bronchus ≤ 2 cm from carina
- T4: involving mediastinum, heart, trachea, esophagus, vertebral body; malignant pleural, or pericardial effusion

Lymph nodes:
- N0: No evidence of regional lymph nodes
- N1: Lymph node metastasis to peribronchial or ipsilateral hilar region
- N2: Metastasis to ipsilateral mediastinal lymph nodes or subcarinal lymph nodes
- N3: Metastasis to any contralateral lymph node group

Metastases:
- M0: No evidence of distant metastasis
- M1: Distant metastasis present

Staging of non–small cell carcinoma, based on TNM classification

Stage IA: T1,N0,M0
Stage IB: T2,N0,M0
Stage IIA: T1,N1,M0
Stage IIB: T2,N1,M0 or T3,N0,M0
Stage IIIA: T3,N1,M0 or T1–3,N2,M0
Stage IIIB: any T,N3,M0 or T4, any N,M0
Stage IV: any T, any N, M1

Classification for small cell carcinoma of lung

Limited disease: Tumor is confined to unilateral hemithorax.
Extended disease: Tumor extends beyond hemithorax, or there is a pleural effusion.

Differential diagnosis

Includes nonlung metastasis (colon, prostate, cervical), tuberculosis, or benign pulmonary nodule. Biopsy will help resolve these possible alternative diagnoses.

P **For non–small cell carcinoma, treat based on stage**
For stages I or II malignancy, order pulmonary function tests (PFTs) to decide if the pt is capable of living with only one lung. If the PFTs indicate a possibility, arrange for surgical resection

This stage of lung cancer is curable. Although only a lobe may need to be resected, pts should be capable of living with only one lung, in case surgical complications require complete resection.

All stage III pts will require chemotherapy and radiation. Stage IIIA may be amenable to surgical resection, whereas stage IIIB will not
Pts with stage IV are incurable and should receive palliative treatment only
For small cell carcinoma, all pts require chemotherapy with a cisplatin/etoposide-based regimen

Use radiation for cerebral metastases, and surgery may be effective for very limited disease. Overall, the prognosis of small cell carcinoma is dismal.

S **Does the pt have any GI symptoms?**
Although pts can present with nonspecific symptoms (e.g., weight loss, anorexia, and
  fatigue) or no symptoms at all, certain symptoms can suggest on which side of the
  colon the cancer is located:
- Anemia and dull vague abdominal pain are associated more with right-sided
  rather than left-sided colon cancers.
- Left-sided colon cancers more typically exhibit constipation, diarrhea, change in
  stool caliber, rectal bleeding, and intestinal obstruction.

Is the pt at any increased risk of developing colon cancer?
Age: Incidence increases after age 45.
Race: Higher incidence exists among African-Americans than whites.
Personal or family history of neoplasm, including benign polyps: Consider more periodic
  screening in these pts.
Inflammatory bowel disease: The cumulative risk can reach up to 20% after 30 years.

O **Perform PE**
Gen: Cachexia can be seen in pts with advanced or long-standing history of carcinoma.
Abd: Advanced disease may present with a palpable abdominal mass or hepatomegaly.
Rectal: A digital rectal examination can reveal mass in about half of rectal cancer cases.
  Stool will often be positive for occult blood on a guaiac card.
Otherwise, most pts will have a normal PE.

Consider ordering the following laboratories
CBC: May present with anemia.
Liver function test: Elevation could signify hepatic metastases.
Carcinoembryonic antigen (CEA): Often elevated in pts with colon cancer. Measure in
  all pts with confirmed colon cancer to monitor treatment.

Obtain a CXR
Although a negative CXR does not rule out metastatic disease, nodules on CXR are
  likely to represent metastases.

Obtain colonoscopy and consider imaging study
Colonoscopy is the diagnostic procedure of choice.
- Allows for biopsy of lesion at the same time as direct visualization.
- If the pt refuses colonoscopy, or for some reason will not tolerate the procedure,
  barium enema and CT colonography can be used in lieu of colonoscopy to detect
  cancers with great reliability.
If biopsy from colonoscopy reveals colon cancer, CT scan of the chest, abdomen, and
  pelvis should be ordered to evaluate for metastases.

A **Carcinoma of the colon**
Be sure to classify the stage of the cancer, because this has implications on treatment and prognosis, and survival.

TNM Classification for colon cancer
Tumor:
- Tis: Carcinoma in situ, confined to epithelium or lamina propria
- T1: Invasion of submucosa
- T2: Invasion of muscularis propria
- T3: Invasion into subserosa or pericolic or perirectal tissue
- T4: Invasion of other organs or structures

Lymph nodes:
- N0: No evidence of regional lymph nodes metastases
- N1: Metastasis in 1 to 3 pericolic or perirectal lymph nodes
- N2: Metastasis in ≥ 4 pericolic or perirectal lymph nodes
- N3: Metastasis in any lymph node along the course of a vascular trunk

Metastases:
- M0: No evidence of distant metastasis
- M1: Distant metastasis present (liver most common, followed by lung)

Staging of colon cancer based on TNM classification
Stage I: T1,N0,M0; T2,N0,M0
Stage II: T3,N0,M0; T4,N0,M0
Stage III: any T,N1–3,M0
Stage IV: M1, any T/N

Differential diagnoses for the symptomatology include
- Inflammatory bowel disease   - Irritable bowel syndrome
- Infectious colitis   - Diverticulosis/diverticulitis

P **Treatment is based on the given stage**
Stage I: Surgical resection of the tumor with end-to-end anastomosis
Stage II: Resection-anastomosis with postoperative adjuvant chemotherapy (5-fluorouracil and leucovorin), radiotherapy, OR immunotherapy.
Stage III: Resection-anastomosis with postoperative adjuvant chemotherapy, radiotherapy, AND immunotherapy.
Stage IV: Chemotherapy for palliative treatment (fluorouracil, leucovorin, and irinotecan). There is no known cure for stage IV disease.

As noted above, after treatment, pts should have CEA levels monitored to rule out recurrence. Elevations in the levels likely means metastatic disease

S

What is the pt's age and ethnicity?
Nearly all pts with prostate cancer are 65 y/o or more. *African Americans tend to be at higher risk than other ethnicities for prostate cancer.*

Does the pt have a father or a brother who has had prostate cancer?
Those with a family history of prostate cancer are also at a higher associated risk.

Are there any symptoms of advanced disease?
Extensive local involvement:

- Dysuria	- Urinary retention	- Increased frequency
- Back pain	- Hematuria	- Outflow obstruction

Metastatic disease:

- Bone pain   - Fractures   - Deep vein thromboses
- Lower extremity weakness (cord compression)   - Pulmonary emboli

More than 80% of pts with prostate cancer are asymptomatic at the time of diagnosis.

O

Perform a PE
Cachexia can be seen in pts with advanced or long-standing history of carcinoma.
Digital rectal exam (DRE) may reveal an enlarged, indurated prostate with focal nodules.
A normal prostate exam does not argue strongly for or against prostate cancer because pts with prostate cancer can have elevated prostate-specific antigen (PSA) and a normal DRE.
Perform a complete neurologic exam of the lower extremities to rule out cord compression.

Obtain a PSA tumor marker test
A normal PSA is less than 4 ng/mL; a value greater than 10 ng/mL has about a 2 in 3 chance of being associated with prostate cancer.

Obtain a transrectal ultrasound of the prostate with or without MRI
Ultrasound findings will help stage the tumor.
Systematic biopsy can be done during ultrasound if malignancy is suspected.
If tissue biopsies confirm prostate cancer, an MRI is the more accurate way to visualize both the prostate and regional lymph node involvement.

Order a radionuclide bone scan to detect any bony metastases
Prostate cancer has a high propensity to metastasize to the bone. It causes what are known as blastic lesions, called that because osteoblastic activity is stimulated. Osteoblasts increase the formation of new bone and thus cause increased uptake of radionuclides.

There is little usefulness in CT scan for staging of prostate cancer

A

Carcinoma of the prostate
Gleason score should be available by pathology
In adenocarcinoma of the prostate, the part of the tumor with the highest histologic grade determines its biologic activity. Higher scores = more likely metastatic disease.
To determine a Gleason score, the pathologist assigns a number to the histologic grade of two areas of the tumor, and each is scored from 1 to 5 (1 is best differentiated, 5 is worst). The two scores are added up to give a Gleason score of 2 to 10.

TNM Classification for prostate cancer

Stage T1: cancer not detectable by DRE
- T1a: with cancer in ≤ 5% of tissue resected, usually found at autopsy or on resection for prostatic hyperplasia
- T1b: with cancer in > 5% of tissue resected, usually found at autopsy or on resection for prostatic hyperplasia
- T1c: cancer found on biopsy indicated by elevated PSA

Stage T2: cancer palpable on DRE but confined to prostate
- T2a: single nodule in only one lobe, surrounded by normal tissue
- T2b: tumor in the majority of one lobe
- T2c: tumor involves both lobes of prostate

Stage T3: palpable tumor extends beyond the prostate without distant metastases
- T3a: unilateral extracapsular extension
- T3b: bilateral extracapsular extension
- T3c: tumor invades seminal vesicles

For all T stages M (metastases) are either (+) or (−).
- M1–2: only pelvic nodes are involved
- M2+: distant metastases

Any T stage can have M+. Metastases can only be diagnosed by pelvic lymphadenectomy.

Approximately 10% of all tumors with a Gleason score < 5 have lymphatic metastases, whereas they exist in 70% of all tumors with scores ≥ 9. However, a PSA of < 10 ng/mL carries only a 10% chance of lymphatic spread. Based on these numbers, a pt and his physician must make the decision to perform a pelvic lymphadenectomy.

P **Refer the pt to a urologist, because surgery is the best hope of cure**

Simple prostatectomy may be curative in T1a and T1c disease.

Radical prostatectomy (removal of prostate and seminal vesicles) improves survival for stages T1b and all of T2.

Radical prostatectomy may be useful in stages T3 with or without M+, in that morbidity from the tumor will likely be reduced. However, benefit on mortality is uncertain.

If the pt refuses surgery or is not a candidate, radiation is a viable option

External-beam radiation is likely to cause impotence (60% of all pts remain sexually functional following surgery).

Radioactive seed implantation seems best suited for T2a disease.

Useful in pts with high-grade malignancies and in pts with positive surgical margins.

For pts with M+ tumor, androgen deprivation tends to slow the rate of growth

Androgen deprivation can be accomplished surgically (castration) or medically. Gonadotropin-releasing hormone antagonists to prevent luteinizing hormone secretion seems to be the preferred method.

Chemotherapy is a last resort for palliation

Only 10% of M+ pts have an objective partial response.

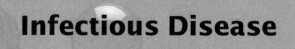

VII

Infectious Disease

S **Does the pt have symptoms that fit the criteria of fever of unknown (FUO)?**

To remember the criteria, remember the number 3.
- Fever should be greater than 101.0°F (38.3°C) for ≥ 3 weeks followed by 3 consecutive days of hospitalization OR 3 outpatient visits without a confirmed diagnosis.

The 3 weeks are not necessary for diagnosis of FUO if the fever begins in a pt already hospitalized for a noninfectious problem (nosocomial FUO), if the pt is neutropenic (neutropenic FUO), or if the pt is HIV positive (HIV-associated FUO).

Does the pt have a history of any autoimmune diseases?
Any autoimmune disease can be associated with others, and these may present with fevers.

Has the pt had any exposure to tuberculosis (TB)?
TB is a common cause of FUO.

Does the pt practice unsafe sex or use injection drugs?
HIV can also cause an FUO.
IV drug usage is also a risk factor for endocarditis, another common cause of FUO.

Does the pt have any history of recent travel?
Third world nations carry a risk of parasitic (e.g., malaria) or chronic bacterial (e.g., brucella) infections.

Has the pt noticed any masses or lumps on the body?
Malignancy is a common cause of FUO. Lumps may represent lymph nodes or tumors.

Is the pt taking any medications?
Many medications can produce fever.

Does the pt have any other physical symptoms that may lead you to a diagnosis?

- Headaches	- Night sweats	- Weight loss
- Anorexia	- Rashes	- Arthritis
- Cough/hemoptysis	- Diarrhea	- Swelling

Ask if the pt is on chronic immunosuppression
If so, consider organisms such as cytomegalovirus, fungi, or *Pneumocystis carinii*.

O **Document the actual severity and frequency of fevers**
This will rule out factitious disorder/malingering and may show a pattern consistent with certain diseases:
- *Two daily spikes*: consistent with Still disease (the systemic form of juvenile rheumatoid arthritis [JRA], which can also occur in adults)
- *Fever every third or fourth day*: consistent with malaria

Conduct a thorough PE to look for any potential causes of the fever
Rash: malar rash of systemic lupus erythematosus, cellulitis, JRA, or polyarteritis nodosa (PAN)
Petechiae: leukemia, endocarditis
Lymphadenopathy: HIV, lymphoma, other malignancy
Systolic murmur: endocarditis
Decreased breath sounds: pneumonia, empyema, TB

RUQ tenderness: liver abscess
Thyromegaly: thyroiditis, Grave's disease (with thyrotoxicosis)

A Fever of Unknown Origin
With criteria as noted above, it is now the practitioner's job to ascertain the actual cause.
- For nosocomial FUOs, note that septic thromboembolism is a common event and that medications may cause fever either on their own or by allowing for opportunistic infections.
- For HIV-associated FUO, seek out opportunistic infections.
- For neutropenic FUO, ascertaining the cause is less important than keeping the pt alive until the neutrophil count recovers.

For a differential diagnosis of all other FUOs (a.k.a. Classic FUO), remember ABCs!

<u>A</u>utoimmune diseases, <u>B</u>ugs (Infections), and <u>C</u>ancer will account for some 60% to 80% of all causes of FUOs. The following are some common diseases that cause fever:

- *Autoimmune*: lupus, JRA, PAN, cryoglobulinemia, polymyalgia rheumatica, Still's disease
- *Bugs* (infections): pneumonia; urinary tract infection; cellulitis; sinusitis; meningitis; endocarditis; abscess of liver, spleen, kidney, or bone; tuberculosis; fungi; HIV; malaria; viral infections
- *Cancer*: Consider solid tumors as well humoral malignancies.
- *Drugs*: steroids, amphetamines, antibiotics, atropine, isoniazid, procainamide, quinidine
- *Endocrine*: hyperthyroidism, thyroiditis
- *Embolism*: deep vein thrombosis or pulmonary embolus
- *Factitious or Familial* Mediterranean fever
- *Granulomatous*: sarcoidosis, Crohn's disease, ulcerative colitis

P Perform cultures on the pt at all sites
Blood cultures times 2, sputum, urine cultures are indicated in all pts with FUO.
Cerebrospinal fluid and peritoneal cultures if relevant.
Be sure to send blood and sputum in special media to look for fungal and TB species if clinical suspicion is raised during history and physical.

Order radiographic studies as clinical suspicion warrants
A CXR should be done on all pts with FUO as part of the initial workup. However, the following studies should only be done based on clinical suspicion:

- KUB	- RUQ ultrasound	- Upper GI series
- CT Chest/Abdomen/Pelvis	- Echocardiography	

Administer empiric antibiotics if the pt appears ill or unstable
Broad-spectrum antibiotics for bacterial infections are a good initial choice. If the pt fails to improve after a few days, consider empiric use of antifungal medicines.
Steroids have not been shown to be of empiric benefit in pts with FUO and may in fact worsen the condition of pts with occult infections.

Send off other serum studies
CBC with differential, antinuclear antibody, rheumatoid factor

Realize that up to 15% cases of FUO resolve or persist without a confirmed diagnosis

S Does the pt have fever, fatigue, muscular pain, or malaise?
These are very general complaints, but these are the common complaints in
endocarditis.

Does the pt have a history of valvular heart disease or rheumatic fever?
Any abnormality of the heart valves increases the risk of endocarditis.
Rheumatic fever (RF) is one of the primary causes of mitral valve stenosis.

Does the pt have a prosthetic heart valve?
Treatment differs considerably based on whether it is a native or prosthetic valve
(see below).

Has the pt ever used IV drugs?
IV drug use is a huge risk factor for endocarditis. It also changes the treatment
approach (see below).

Does the pt report any new dyspnea on exertion or decreased exercise
tolerance?
Congestive heart failure resulting from valvular disease is one of the sequelae of
endocarditis, as well as a reason to consider surgery as a treatment option.

O Review VS and perform a PE
Look for fever (temperature $> 100.4°F = 38°C$)
Neuro: defects as a sign of possible stroke from septic emboli
Cardio: murmur, especially one consistent with valvular regurgitation
HEENT: Roth spots (round white spots surrounded by a retinal hemorrhage)
Skin:
  • *Janeway lesions*: painless hemorrhagic macules/nodules on the palms, soles
  • *Osler nodes*: painful pea-sized subcutaneous nodules in the fingers, toes, palms,
    soles

Obtain serial blood cultures
These are necessary not only to help make the diagnosis but also to decide on treatment.

Review the CBC with differential
Look for clues suggesting bacterial infection, such as high white count with left shift.

Check U/A for signs of hematuria or RBC casts
Glomerulonephritis is a well-known immunologic effect of endocarditis.

Order rheumatoid factor
Helps to make the diagnosis because it is one of the minor criteria.

Review the echocardiogram
Look for signs of intracardiac mass, abscess, or other abnormalities, particularly
around a valve.

If transthoracic echo is negative or inconclusive, consider
transesophageal
Often a better view of the heart can be obtained using transesophageal, but it is more
invasive and requires sedation, so it should only be used if transthoracic echo is
inconclusive and clinical suspicion of endocarditis remains high.

Acute Bacterial Endocarditis
Bacterial infection of the inner wall (endocardium) of the heart
Diagnosis is often made using Duke criteria:
- Major Criteria
  1. Two or more positive blood cultures
  2. New murmur or echocardiogram showing endocardial involvement
- Minor Criteria
  1. History of previous valvular abnormality, heart surgery, or IV drug use
  2. Fever
  3. Evidence of septic emboli
  4. Immunologic signs: glomerulonephritis, RF positive, Osler nodes, Roth spots
  5. Single positive blood culture
For diagnosis, you need 2 major or 1 major and 3 minor or 5 minor
For possible endocarditis, you need 1 major and 1 minor or 3 minor

Differential diagnosis
Vasculitis: PAN, MPA, Wegener's disease, HSP
Infectious: meningitis, sepsis, pneumonia, myocarditis, pericarditis, malaria, HIV, syphilis, EBV, CMV
Oncologic: perineoplastic syndrome, metastases
Endocrine: hyperthyroid, hypothyroid, DKA
Rheumatic: SLE, RA, MCTD, JRA

This disease can be subtle, so using the Duke criteria can be helpful in determining the likelihood that this is endocarditis

P **Draw blood cultures and treat first empirically and then based on sensitivities**
Vancomycin with gentamicin is a good choice for empiric treatment.
Duration of treatment is usually about 6 weeks.

Consult Cardiothoracic Surgery for possible surgery if pt has congestive heart failure, abscess, or failure of antibiotics
In these cases, surgery may be the only option.

Consider consulting Cardiology and Infectious Disease for more advice
Advice from the experts is an important component of care. This can be a difficult disease to treat, and even if treated correctly, more than half of these pts require valve replacement eventually.

Provide prophylaxis with amoxicillin or clindamycin 1 hr before invasive procedures like dental procedures
If the pt is high risk and will undergo GI or GU surgery, give IV/IM ampicillin and gentamicin.

S **What is the pt's last CD4 count and viral load?**
Infections like *Pneumocystis carinii* pneumonia (PCP), Cocci, and cytomegalovirus are more common with lower CD4 counts.

Does the pt have a history of opportunistic infections?
Previous PCP infection increases the risk of recurrence.
Examples of organisms that cause opportunistic infection are as follows:
- Fungal (candida, histoplasma, cryptococcus, coccidioides, aspergillus)
- Protozoal/fungal (*pneumocystis carinii*), protozoa (cryptosporidia, microsporidia, isospora), and sporozoa (toxoplasma).

Does the pt have risk factors for exposure to known infection?
Sick contacts: TB exposure, homelessness, incarceration, IV drug abuse
Recent travel: Southwest United States, Arizona (cocci); Ohio/Mississippi river valleys (histo)
Employment: farmers: aspergillus; hunters: blastomycosis
Animal contacts: bird droppings (crypto); cats (toxo); bat droppings (histo)

What medications is the pt taking? Is he or she on HAART or prophylaxis?
If the pt is on TMP/SMX or azithromycin prophylaxis, for example, he or she is less likely to have PCP or membrane attack complex (MAC), respectively.

Does the pt have symptoms suggestive of infection?
CNS: changes in mental status, headache, neck stiffness, and fever (meningitis)
- HIV pts do not have typical symptoms, may be subtle: fatigue and fever.

Respiratory symptoms such as cough, exertional dyspnea, pleuritic chest pain, night sweats, and fever may reflect conditions like sinusitis, bronchitis, and pneumonia. As CD4 counts decrease, PCP, TB, fungal, lymphoma, or Kaposi's sarcoma (KS).
GI symptoms include odynophagia or dysphagia suggesting esophagitis; abdominal pain, diarrhea, and fever suggesting infectious etiology.

O **Review VS, looking for signs of hemodynamic instability**
Sepsis: fever, hypotension, tachycardia
Dehydration: positive orthostatics
Pneumonia: increased respiratory rate, low pulse oximetry

Perform a PE
Gen: assess level of consciousness, nutritional status
HEENT: funduscopic, ulcers, thrush, meningismus, lymph nodes
Abd: hepatomegaly, splenomegaly (histo, TB)
Skin: subcutaneous nodules, ulcers

Evaluate CBC with differential
Leukocytosis with left shift suggests infection; consider urine, blood, sputum, stool cultures, lumbar puncture (LP), and CXR (cultures should include bacteria, fungal, and acid-fast bacillus [AFB]).
Anemia (chronic disease, parvovirus B-19) also occurs often.
Thrombocytopenia: common in HIV

Obtain a CD4 count
Some infections are more common at lower CD4 counts:
- CD4 > 500 cells/mm^3: sinusitis, bronchitis, oral thrush
- CD4 200–500 cells/mm^3: pneumonia (bacterial)

- CD4 100–200 cells/mm^3: PCP, histo, cocci, miliary TB, lymphoma
- CD4 < 100 cells/mm^3: toxo, crypto, MAC, KS
- CD4 < 50 cells/mm^3: CMV infections

Consider further diagnostic studies

If predominant CNS symptoms, consider:
- CT head: Ring-enhancing lesions suggest toxoplasma or lymphoma.
- LP: opening pressure, cell count, protein, glucose, Gram stain, culture, AFB, VDRL test, cryptococcal Ag
- Serum crypto Ag, toxoplasma Ab

If predominant pulmonary symptoms, consider:
- Sputum Gram stain, cx: fungal, AFB, PCP (expectorated or induced)
- Place purified protein derivative (PPD)
- LDH: increased with PCP, TB, lymphoma
- ABG: hypoxemia and high A-a gradient common with PCP
- CXR: Normal CXR does not indicate absence of disease.
  - Bilateral interstitial infiltrates common with PCP, histo, cocci
  - Upper lobe cavitary lesion with TB or pentamidine treated PCP
  - Pleural effusions common with TB or KS
- Consider CT chest or bronchoscopy

If predominant GI symptoms, consider:
- Send stool WBC, culture, ova and parasites, isospora and cryptospora

If any suspicious skin lesions, biopsy

HIV and Fever

Infection in HIV-positive pts requires special consideration because they are immunosuppressed and therefore at increased risk from not only normal pathogens but also a wide range of opportunistic infections.

Etiologies

CNS infections (*S. pneumoniae*, crypto, HSV, VSV, toxo)
Pulmonary infections (*S. pneum.*, *H. influenzae*, TB, PCP, *Rhodococcus equi*)
GI infections (candida, HSV, CMV, crypto-/iso-/microspora, MAC)
Malignancy (lymphoma, KS, cervical or anal cancer)

Ensure that the pt is on appropriate prophylaxis

If CD4 count < 200, start PCP prophylaxis with TMP/SMX.
If CD4 count < 100, start MAC prophylaxis with azithromycin.

Treat based on source of infection

Esophagitis: fluconazole (candida)
Sinusitis or bronchitis: amoxicillin or augmentin
TB: (see TB, p. 20)
MAC: clarithromycin 500 mg twice per day
PCP: TMP/SMZ DS (or pentamadine if allergic) for 21 days
- If PaO$_2$ < 70, a-A gradient > 35, give steroids.
- Lifelong prophylactic therapy with TMP/SMZ DS or dapsone if allergic

Cryptococcal meningitis: amphotericin B
Histoplasmosis: mild-moderate disease: itraconazole; severe disease: amphotericin B
- Maintenance therapy: itraconazole

Coccidioidomycosis or aspergillosis: amphotericin B
Toxoplasmosis: pyramethamine and sulfadiazine

S **Does the pt report any recent breaks in the skin?**
Many things can cause a break in the skin and be a portal of entry for infection:

- Abrasions	- Cuts	- Burns
- Bites (insect, dog, cat)	- Surgical wound	- IVs
- IV drug abuse (IVDA)	- Preexisting skin conditions	

Does the pt have any preexisting skin problems?
These conditions can also cause a break in the skin and lead to cellulitis:

- Eczema	- Psoriasis	- Pemphigus
- Athlete's foot	- Venous stasis	- Pressure ulcer

Does the pt have diabetes?
Increased risk, especially in poorly controlled diabetes mellitus:
- Poor immune system activity, especially with hyperglycemia
- Decreased peripheral sensation, may not notice foot injuries like stepping on a piece of glass

Is the pt using IV drugs or skin popping?
Intravenous or subcutaneous use of drugs or other substances is another risk factor for infection.

Is the pt homeless or alcoholic?
These pts tend to be at increased risk for skin infection resulting from poor hygiene.

Does the pt have any other medical problems?
Renal failure, especially end-stage renal failure, also leads to poor healing and increased risk of cellulitis and other infections.
Similarly, hepatic failure/cirrhosis can lead to poor healing.
Malnutrition from any cause can lead to poor healing.
Pts with cancer have an increased risk from things like chemotherapy, which can weaken the immune system, to central venous catheters, which can be portals of entry for the infection.

Review the medicines the pt is taking
It is important to note immune-suppressing medicines like prednisone.

Does the pt have any other preexisting immune deficiency?
Neutrophil (both acquired and congenital) defects like neutropenia and chronic granulomatous disease (CGD) place the pt at particularly increased risk.
HIV can also lead to immune deficiency and a variety of opportunistic infections.

O **Review the VS and perform a PE**
Look for fever, which may indicate infection with *Staphylococcus pyogenes* or that there is more than cellulitis: abscess, toxic shock syndrome, endocarditis.
Skin:
- Look specifically at the lesion for redness, warmth, swelling, and pain.
- Note if the cellulitis overlies any bones or joints.
- Palpate carefully for any crepitus or fluctuance.
- Look for signs of underlying trauma, such as:

- Abrasion	- Bites	- Burns	- Cuts

- Look for signs of underlying skin disease, such as:

- Tinea	- Herpes	- Eczema
- Folliculitis	- Venous stasis	- Pressure ulcers

Look in the ear, especially in diabetics who are prone to infections like otitis externa.
Examine the lower leg (one of the most common sites).

Ask IV drug abusers to show you where they inject.
Feel for lymph nodes in the area.

Consider biopsy/culture of the inflamed skin
This may give you the diagnosis as well as the best treatment if you can get sensitivities
from the culture.

Consider obtaining an x-ray or MRI if the lesion overlies superficial bone
Look for signs of periosteal elevation suggesting osteomyelitis.

A Cellulitis
Acute inflammation of the skin caused by bacterial infection leading to warmth,
redness, swelling, and local pain.

Etiologies
Staphlylococcus aureus: usually spreads from a local infection like an abscess caused by a
foreign body. Associated with IVDA. Consider possible endocarditis.
Streptococcus pyogenes: usually diffuse and rapidly spreading associated with
lymphangitis as well as fever
Streptococcal (groups A,B, C, or G): associated with venous stasis/peripheral vascular
disease and pts with diabetes
Haemophilus influenzae: associated with infections above the neck (sinusitis, otitis) and
people with diabetes
Pseudomonas aeruginosa: diabetics, hot tub folliculitis, and people who step on a nail
while wearing tennis shoes
Pasteurella multocida: associated with cat and dog bites
Vibrio vulnificus: associated with shell fish/ocean
Mycobacterium marinarum: associated with fish tanks and swimming pools

Differential diagnosis
- Necrotizing fasciitis	- Gangrene	- Herpes
- Osteomyelitis	- Eczema	- Viral exanthem
- Folliculitis	- Abscess	- Tinea
- Elder abuse	- Burn	- Endocarditis
- Toxic shock syndrome	- Lyme disease	- HIV
- Mucormycosis	- Cryptococcus	- CGD

P In general, empiric therapy can begin with Keflex or oxacillin
These drugs will cover most of the common causes of cellulitis (Group A Strep and
Staph aureus).

If empiric therapy fails or the pt has an underlying immunodeficiency, consider admission for IV antibiotics
If the pt fails outpatient empiric therapy, then he or she may have:
- Unidentified immune deficiency (HIV, ESRD, cancer)
- MRSA or other resistant organisms: Admit for IV vancomycin.
- Osteomyelitis, endocarditis, or other underlying infections/conditions
- Diabetes: Make sure there is good anaerobic coverage because of the increased
risk of anaerobic coinfection.

Carefully identify pts who need surgical intervention
Some pts may need surgical debridement:
       - Necrotizing fasciitis   - Abscess   - Pyomyositis
Pts with osteomyelitis will need Orthopedic consultation.

Consult Dermatology in cases that are not clear

VIII

Endocrinology

S **Does the pt have any risk factors for diabetes?**
          - Obesity   - Polycystic ovarian syndrome   - Gestational diabetes
Multiple first-degree relatives with diabetes
   • Type 1 DM associated with HLA-DR3 or HLA-DR4
Ethnicity
   • Type 1 DM: Scandinavians are highest risk
   • Type 2 DM: African-Americans, Mexicans, Native Americans

What is the pt's age?
Type 1 DM is common in children 10 to 14 years of age or in older nonobese pts.
Type 2 DM is common in those older than 40 years of age.

Does the pt experience the 3 P's (polyuria, polydipsia, polyphagia)?
Type 1 DM often presents with polyuria and weight loss.

O **Review VS**
Obesity (BMI > 30), calculate using: BMI = (Wt in kg)/(Ht in m)^2.
   • So a 100-kg (220-lb) person who is 1.83 m (72 inches or 6 ft) tall has a BMI of:
      $100/(1.83)^2 = 29.8$.
High blood pressure (risk for micro and macrovascular complications)
Orthostatics (assess volume status)

Perform a complete PE, looking specifically for
Gen: Assess mental status.
HEENT: Perform a funduscopic exam; inspect dentition.
Ext: Document integrity of skin, edema or deformities, strength of pulses.
Neuro: Assess sensation using monofilament if possible.

Review renal function tests
Obtain creatinine to assess renal impairment. Some medications like metformin (if
   Cr > 1.6 men or > 1.5 women) are contraindicated in this case.

Perform diagnostic test
Criteria for diagnosing DM include:
   • Random blood sugar (BS) > 200 mg/dL (two separate occasions)
      ◆ 110–200 mg/dL = impaired glucose tolerance
   • Fasting blood sugar (FBS) > 126 mg/dL (two separate occasions)
      ◆ 110–126 mg/dL = impaired glucose tolerance
   • 2-hour plasma glucose > 200 mg/dL (oral glucose tolerance test, OGTT)
      ◆ 140–200 mg/dL = impaired glucose tolerance

Check HbA1c
Typically, RBCs live about 110 days in the blood stream, and during that time they can
   become glycated. For this reason, this test can be used to estimate the level of glycemic
   control in the last approximately 3 months. Normal HbA1c is 6.
You can calculate a corresponding BS using the HbA1c:
   • Average BS = [(HbA1c – 4)35] + 65
   • So HbA1c of 7 = avg BS of = [(7 – 4)35] + 65 = 170

Review results of a fasting lipid panel
Pts commonly have triglycerides > 200 mg/dL and HDL < 35 mg/dL

Check Urinalysis
Glucosuria occurs when the threshold for reabsorption of glucose is exceeded.
Ketonuria suggests diabetic ketoacidosis (DKA) or starvation.
Send urine specifically for microalbumin.

Look for evidence of the metabolic syndrome
Pts with metabolic syndrome have a higher prevalence of coronary artery disease.
The metabolic syndrome is defined by the presence of three or more of the following:
- Obesity: waist circumference > 40 inches in men, > 35 inches in women
- Dyslipidemia:
  - ◆ Fasting triglycerides > 150 mg/dL
  - ◆ HDL cholesterol < 40 mg/dL in men, < 50 mg/dL in women
- Hypertension: blood pressure > 130/85 mm Hg
- Diabetes: fasting plasma glucose > 110 mg/dL

A Diabetes Mellitus
Type 2 Diabetes: poor glycemic control resulting from insulin resistance and decreased
   insulin secretion in response to hyperglycemia
Type 1 Diabetes: poor glycemic control resulting from absence of endogenous insulin
   secretion (> 90% autoimmune)
Secondary Diabetes
   - Pancreatic disorders   - Genetic (hemochromatosis)
   - Cushing's syndrome   - Drugs (steroids)

P Identify and treat pts with DKA/HONK (see p. 128)
Educate all pts before initiating medications
Diabetic teaching (e.g., pathophysiology, complications, lifestyle)
Glucometer for home glucose monitoring
Log of adverse effects, especially of symptoms such as sweating, tremulousness, and
   confusion because these may be a sign of overmedication
Nutrition, exercise, smoking cessation, immunizations (pneumococcal, influenza)

Keep treatment goals in mind at each visit
   - HbA1c < 6.5%   - LDL < 100 mg/dL   - Blood pressure
   - HDL > 40 mg/dL   - Triglycerides < 150 mg/dL   < 130/80 mm Hg

Begin with oral medications like biguanides or sulfonylurea
Begin with monotherapy and then a combination of oral agents before insulin.
   - Sulfonylureas (glyburide,   - Thiazolidinediones
     glipizide)   (rosiglitazone)
   - Biguanides (metformin)   - α-glucosidase inhibitors
   - Combination (glyburide/   (acarbose)
     metformin)

Begin insulin if pt fails to reach goals with oral medications
In general, the amount of insulin can be estimated based on the pt's weight. Use about
0.6 per kg to estimate the units needed, and then use two-thirds in the morning and
one-third in the evening. Of the morning dose, two-thirds should be intermediate
and one-third short-acting. In the evening, use one-half intermediate and one-half
short-acting.
   - Ultra-short-acting (lispro, aspart)   - Intermediate (NPH, lente)
   - Short-acting (Novolin, Humulin, regular)   - Long-acting (glargine)
   - Mixed combinations (70/30, 50/50)

Refer pt annually to Ophthalmology, Dentistry, and Podiatry
Such referrals will help reduce the number of complications, such as blindness, tooth
loss, and amputation.

S What is the pt's age?

Certain age groups are more likely to present with DKA versus HONK.
- DKA is common in young type 1 DM, also seen with type 2.
- HONK is common in older pts, seen in type 2.

Does the pt report any of the 3 P's (polyuria, polydipsia, polyphagia)?

Common clinical manifestations of uncontrolled hyperglycemia:
- Polyuria: frequent urination caused by glycosuria
- Polydipsia: frequent drinking driven by dehydration and hyperosmolarity
- Polyphagia: increased food intake often with weight loss

Does the pt report recent illness?

Decompensated glycemic control results from underlying infections
- Urinary tract infection   - Pneumonia   - Pancreatitis

Other factors that may precipitate hyperglycemia
- Myocardial infarction (MI)   - Cerebrovascular accident
- Alcohol binge   - Pregnancy   - Trauma

Does the pt have a history of lack of adherence to medications or nutrition?

Nonadherence is one of the most common causes of poorly controlled sugars.

Review medications

Diuretics and steroids can increase blood sugars.

O Does the pt have VS suggestive of hemodynamic instability?

Consider the following in a pt who presents with severe hyperglycemia:
- *Sepsis*: fever, hypotension, tachycardia
- *Respiratory distress*: tachypnea (Kussmaul respirations)
- *Severe volume contraction*: orthostatics

Perform a PE

Gen: Assess level of consciousness (obtunded); evaluate for acetone breath.
Look for signs of infection.

Perform diagnostic tests to differentiate DKA from HONK

Check finger stick.
Check arterial blood gas (ABG).
- Low pH in DKA, normal in HONK

Check serum electrolytes, including calcium, magnesium, and phosphorus.
- Calculate anion gap.
  - ◆ High in DKA, normal in HONK

Check serum ketones.
- High in DKA, none/decreased in HONK

Calculate serum osmolality: increased in HONK.
- $2 \times$ (observed $Na^+ + K^+$) + glucose/18 + BUN/2.8

What is the result of the CBC with differential?

Leukocytosis with left shift indicates infection.
- Consider U/A, blood, urine and sputum cultures, and CXR.

What are the results of the pt's renal and liver function tests (LFTs)?

Pts who are severely volume contracted typically have a rise in BUN and creatinine.
Abnormal LFTs suggest infection or alcohol-induced.

Consider the ECG
MI is a common precipitant of a severe hyperglycemic state.
Arrhythmias are common with electrolyte abnormalities.

Severe Hyperglycemia
Diabetic Ketoacidosis
- DM: *hyperglycemia (glucose > 300 mg/dL)*
- *Ketonuria, ketonemia, or both*
- *Acidosis pH < 7.35, bicarbonate < 15*

Hyperosmolar Nonketotic Coma
- Hyperglycemia (glucose > 400 mg/dL)
- Impaired mental status
- High plasma osmolality (> 340 mOsm)
- Lack of significant ketosis

Admit to a monitored bed
DKA and HONK are life-threatening conditions.

Treat precipitating factors
As mentioned above, many things can cause or precipitate DKA/HONK; look for these
causes and treat them or the pt will not get better.

Provide aggressive fluid resuscitation immediately, even before insulin
These pts (HONK > DKA) are very volume depleted.
Estimated free water deficit = $0.5 \times$ body wt (kg) $\times$ (corrected Na^+-140/140)
Initial volume replacement with normal saline (NS). Replace 1 L in first hour, 2nd L in
next 1 to 2 hours, and then continue 1/2NS 500 mL/hr.

Add D5 to IV fluid when glucose levels approach 250 mg/dL
To avoid rebound hypoglycemia

IV insulin therapy: load 0.1 to 0.2 U/kg IV and then continuous infusion 0.1U/kg/hr
This will decrease serum glucose concentration.
Continue until anion gap $[AG = Na - (Cl + HCO_3)]$ is closed (AG < 15).
SQ dose of regular insulin 30 minutes before stopping infusion

Make a flow sheet of important electrolytes and glucose to carefully follow and replace electrolytes
In hyperosmolar states, the electrolytes K, Ca, Mg, and Phos will be artificially high in
the serum because of the lack of insulin. So it is important to monitor them carefully
in order to avoid dangerous sequelae of low serum electrolytes (such as arrhythmia)
as the insulin is replaced.

Finger sticks every hour initially
Carefully avoid hypoglycemia (remember to add D5 when the blood sugar approaches
250) and make sure your interventions are working.

Electrolytes, anion gap q2 hrs initially. P, Mg q6 hrs initially
As mentioned above, treatment is not over until AG < 15, and these pts will nearly
always require electrolyte replacement.

Repeat ABG after 4 hrs
Another way of verifying that your interventions are working.

S Does the pt experience symptoms related to a hypothyroid state?
- Fatigue   - Weakness   - Cold intolerance   - Weight gain
- Constipation   - Dyspnea   - Brittle hair/nails   - Dry skin
- Muscle cramps - Depression   - Difficulty concentrating
- Loss of hearing (fluid accumulation in middle ear)

Does the female pt report changes in her menstrual cycle?
Evaluate thyroid function with any menstrual irregularity or history of infertility.

Does the pt have a history of Graves' disease?
Previous radioablation and thyroidectomy are risks for primary hypothyroidism.

Does the pt have risk factors for central hypothyroidism?
Pts with central nervous system (CNS) lesions are at risk for a hypothyroid state.
- Head trauma   - Pituitary tumors   - CNS radiation

Does the pt have symptoms associated with other pituitary hormones?
Consider other hormones of pituitary gland as being affected:
- Stunted growth (growth hormone)
- Hypogonadism, dysmenorrhea (FSH/LH)
- Decreased libido/lactation (prolactin)

Does the pt have a history of autoimmune disease?
- Pernicious anemia   - Type 1 diabetes mellitus
- Myasthenia gravis   - Vitiligo

Does the pt have a history of infiltrative disease?
Places pt at risk for developing hypothyroidism:
- Hemochromatosis   - Sarcoidosis   - Amyloidosis

Review medications
Medications may affect thyroid hormone secretion or metabolism.
- Propylthiouracil   - Methimazole   - Lithium   - Amiodarone

O Review the pt's VS for signs of hypothyroidism
- Bradycardia   - Diastolic hypertension   - Hypothermia

Perform PE
Gen: assess level of consciousness
HEENT: alopecia, periorbital edema, thinning outer eyebrow, goiter, hoarseness
Skin: nonpitting edema (myxedema), dryness, pallor
Ext: cool to touch
Neuro: delayed relaxation of deep tendon reflexes

Review CBC and renal function
Abnormal lipids may affect RBC morphology, causing macrocytic anemia.
Pts with elevated BUN and creatinine suggests volume contraction.

Evaluate the pattern of TSH and thyroid hormone
Elevated TSH, decreased free T4 (primary hypothyroidism)
Decreased or normal TSH, decreased free T4 (central hypothyroidism)
Elevated TSH, normal free T4, T3 (subclinical hypothyroidism)

Consider antithyroid peroxidase or antithyroglobulin
Obtain antibodies in a pt suspected of autoimmune disease: subclinical
  hypothyroidism with positive antibodies have a 4% risk of hypothyroidism.

Hypothyroidism
Inadequate secretion of thyroid hormone

Etiologies
Primary (Thyroid):
- Hashimoto thyroiditis   - Radiation   - Thyroidectomy
- Subacute thyroiditis   - Drugs   - Iodine excess
- Iodine deficiency   - Congenital
Secondary (Pituitary):
- Tumor   - Infiltrative disease   - Sheehan (postpartum)
Tertiary (Hypothalamic):
- Tumor   - Radiation   - Infection

Identify pts with myxedema coma
A pt who presents with altered level of consciousness, hypothermia, hypoxia, bradycardia, and hypotension with known hypothyroidism must be treated promptly!

P **Myxedema coma is a medical emergency**
Admit to monitored bed.
Load L-thyroxine 400 µg IV, then 100 µg IV qd.

Avoid aggressive rewarming
Causes vasodilation worsening hypertension
Respiratory support may be needed because of decompensation with shock and coma.

Support respiratory status as needed.
Look for precipitating cause
- Infection   - GI bleed   - Congestive heart failure
- Myocardial infarction   - Cerebrovascular accident   - Trauma

Have low threshold for starting IV antibiotics
Check cortisol level and replace as needed
Identify pts with thyroiditis and treat them symptomatically
Pts with thyroiditis usually do not require hormone replacement. Monitoring and symptomatic care is sufficient because this condition is usually self-limited.

Identify primary hypothyroidism and treat with L-thyroxine 1.7 µg/kg/day
- Older pts and those with coronary artery disease should start at lower doses.
- Titrate slowly until TSH is normal, and then reevaluate in 6 to 8 weeks.
- Increase dose with pregnancy.
- Many drug–drug interactions require higher doses.

Identify central hypothyroidism and monitor free T4 levels
This is to assess adrenal function because replacement therapy may precipitate an adrenal crisis.

Subclinical hypothyroidism is usually monitored and not treated
Treatment is controversial; some indications include dyslipidemia or pregnancy.

S **Is the pt experiencing any symptoms of hyperthyroidism?**
Most pts with hyperthyroidism are symptomatic. Common symptoms include:

- Tremors   - Heat intolerance   - Diaphoresis
- Anxiety   - Weight loss   - Diarrhea

Pts older than 70 may not manifest the same typical symptoms as younger pts;
common clinical manifestations in those older than 70 include:

- Atrial fibrillation   - Congestive heart failure (CHF)   - Wasting
- Anorexia   - Fatigue

Has the pt had any fevers?
Rarely, low-grade fevers may occur.

Ask women about changes in their menstrual cycles
Common manifestations include oligomenorrhea and amenorrhea.

Has the pt noticed any weakness?
Often, despite having increased energy, pts could have trouble climbing stairs,
secondary to proximal muscle weakness.

Other than weight loss, has the pt noticed any physical changes?
Goiter might be the most common physical change.
Pts may complain of eye enlargement or a "bug-eyed" appearance. This is known as
exophthalmos or proptosis and is common in Graves' disease.
Some pts may complain about changes of the skin on their shins. It may be thickened,
hyperpigmented, and itchy. This is dermopathy, a myxedema also associated with
Graves' disease.

Is there a family history of thyroid disease?
Family histories of hypo- and hyperthyroidism are common.

O **Review VS**
Low-grade fever may be present. Temperature $> 41°C$ is a sign of thyroid storm.
Tachycardia, increased pulse pressure (high systolic, low diastolic) are common.

Perform a PE
Gen: Wasting, fidgeting, and pressured speech are common.
  • Note if the pt has altered mental status. This is a sign of thyroid storm.
Eyes: Many common findings may occur.
  • Exophthalmos: Common but only occurs in Graves' disease.
  • Staring, lid lag, and lid retraction may occur with all types of hyperthyroidism.
Neck: These pts will likely have a goiter.
  • Diffusely enlarged, smooth, nontender: think Graves' disease.
  • Nodular: Think toxic multinodular goiter versus malignancy.
    ◆ Auscultate over a goiter for a bruit; also common in Graves' disease.
Cardiac: Atrial fibrillation is extremely common; systolic murmurs, signs of CHF
Neuro: A fine tremor is extremely common.
Skin: Commonly, skin will be warm, smooth, and moist. Look for pretibial myxedema
with an orange-skin appearance. Pts may also have vitiligo.

**Send serum for thyroid-stimulating hormone (TSH), free T4, and
T3 levels**
TSH is the most sensitive test for screening. Low in the presence of hyperthyroidism.
High free T4 classical, but some pts will have T3 toxicosis.

**Order thyroid radioiodine uptake if you cannot delineate the etiology
by H&P**
High uptake, homogenous distribution suggests Graves' disease.

Low uptake suggests thyroiditis.
Patchy areas of increased and decreased uptake suggests multinodular goiter.

Obtain an ECG
This will rule out atrial fibrillation.

Hyperthyroidism (thyrotoxicosis)
A syndrome of increased metabolic rate secondary to overproduction of thyroid
  hormone

Differential diagnosis
Graves' disease (most common): an autoimmune condition resulting in an antibody
  that, instead of destroying thyroid tissue, binds to the TSH receptor and stimulates it.
Toxic multinodular goiter: happens in pts who have had long-standing simple goiter.
  More common in the elderly.
Thyroiditis (subacute, painless): an autoimmune condition in which thyroid tissue is
  destroyed. May be a precursor to Hashimoto's thyroiditis or may be self-limiting.
Hyperfunctioning thyroid malignancy: Cancer should always be ruled out by biopsy.

Identify pts with thyroid storm
Pts have a high mortality rate. Admit to a monitored setting immediately!
Identify and treat precipitating factors (usually infection or dehydration):
- Methimazole or propylthiouracil   - Propranolol IV
- Iodide (Lugol's solution)   - Hydrocortisone

Identify pts with thyroiditis
In these pts, there is no role for antithyroid medications or radioactive iodine (RAI)
  because the hyperthyroidism is caused by release of preformed thyroid hormone and
  not overproduction.
Generally resolves spontaneously after 2 to 4 months.

Hyperadrenergic symptoms can be treated with β-blockers
Oral propranolol is the drug of choice.

Excessive thyroid secretion can be treated with antithyroid drugs
Methimazole or propylthiouracil
Monitor for potential side effects: agranulocytosis, hepatitis, lupus-like syndrome.

Indications for radioiodine ablation therapy
Adverse reaction to oral medications
Severe cardiac manifestations
Toxic multinodular goiter
Contraindications: pregnancy, breastfeeding

Indications for subtotal thyroidectomy
Pregnant pts or children with adverse reaction to oral medications
Large goiters with compressive complications

Monitor treatment by following free T4 levels
If the pt has atrial fibrillation or CHF, treat as noted in SOAPs on these illnesses
Refer pts with exophthalmos to Ophthalmology. Orbital radiation may be necessary

S **Does the pt have symptoms associated with hypercalcemia?**
- Fatigue   - Weakness   - Lethargy   - Polyuria   - AMS
- Nausea   - Vomiting   - Constipation - Polydipsia

Review medications
Thiazide diuretics may exacerbate underlying hyperparathyroidism.
Long-term lithium may also cause hyperparathyroidism.

Does the pt have recurrent UTI or kidney stones?
Hyperparathyroidism increases the risk for calcium-containing stones because of the
  increased filtered load of calcium by kidney.

Does the pt have joint pain?
Oligo- or polyarticular pain may suggest underlying pseudogout or gout.

Is there a family history of similar symptoms?
MEN type I: primary hyperparathyroidism, pituitary adenoma, ZE
MEN type IIa: primary hyperparathyroidism, medullary thyroid carcinoma and
  pheochromocytoma
Familial hypocalciuric hypercalcemia (FHH)

O **Review VS**
Hypertension is commonly associated with hyperparathyroidism.

Perform a PE
Gen: Assess level of consciousness.   *Skin*: vitiligo
HEENT: slit lamp (corneal calcifications)   *Ext*: joint effusions
Neuro: proximal muscle weakness

Review CBC and BUN/Cr
Leukocytosis suggests infection (UTI).
Assess for ARF (increased BUN/Cr) caused by UTI, dehydration, or calculi.
  • Consider urinalysis to assess presence of hematuria or pyuria.
  • Consider abdominal film and then renal ultrasound to rule out calculi.

Check total calcium, albumin, or serum ionized calcium
Majority of calcium bound to albumin, correct for changes in serum albumin
  • Corrected Calcium $= [(4.0 - \text{Alb}) \times 0.8] + \text{Measured Calcium.}$

**To rule out possible lab error, consider checking an arterial blood gas
for ionized calcium**
Serum ionized calcium levels are most indicative of actual serum calcium levels.

Check parathyroid hormone (PTH) level to assess gland function
PTH high, calcium high indicates primary hyperparathyroidism.
PTH normal, calcium high suggests primary hyperparathyroidism.
PTH high, calcium low suggests secondary hyperparathyroidism.
PTH low, undetectable, look for another cause of hypercalcemia.

Check phosphate, alkaline phosphatase
PTH increases renal excretion of phosphate, causing low serum phosphate.
PTH increases osteoblast activity, causing high alkaline phosphatase.

Consider 24-hour urine collection for calcium
Increased with primary hyperparathyroidism
  • Men > 300 mg/24 hr; women > 250 mg/24 hr
  • Decreased excretion indicates FHH (< 150 mg/24 hr)

Consider a DEXA scan (see Osteoporosis, p. 140) to rule out osteoporosis
Consider ECG
Hypercalcemia increases risk for arrhythmia or sudden death; look for short QT.

Hyperparathyroidism
Condition in which there is increased secretion of PTH or PTHrP, leading to increased serum calcium, decreased serum phosphorus, and increased excretion of both in the urine. This can lead to urinary calcium stones as well as bone demineralization.

Etiologies
Primary hyperparathyroidism
- Parathyroid adenoma
- Parathyroid carcinoma
- Parathyroid hyperplasia
- MEN Type 1 or IIa

Secondary hyperparathyroidism
- Chronic renal failure

Tertiary hyperparathyroidism
- FHH
- Postrenal transplant

Differential diagnosis
Malignancy (PTHrP), multiple myeloma, iatrogenic, renal failure

Admit pts with symptomatic hypercalcemia
Pts with hyperparathyroidism are at risk for severe increases in calcium (> 12 mg/dL). With severe hypercalcemia, pts are at risk for seizure, arrhythmia, and sudden death.

Administer aggressive IV fluid resuscitation if pt has symptomatic hypercalcemia
Use caution with elderly, cardiac, or renal pts.
Increased serum calcium often causes a diuresis, and on admission many of these pts are intravascularly depleted.
Aggressive fluid hydration also helps reduce the serum calcium by dilution.

Give loop diuretics once the pt is euvolemic
The loop diuretic like furosemide will increase excretion of calcium.

Give calcitonin and bisphosphonates if aggressive IV fluids or loop diuretics are contraindicated or not working
Works at the level of the bone rather than the kidneys to reduce the serum calcium.

Educate pts to avoid dehydration, diuretics, and excess calcium
Monitor asymptomatic pts closely
Every 6 to 12 months calcium, PTH, renal function measurements, and DEXA scan
Surgical indications include:
- Calcium > 11.5 mg/dL or episode of life-threatening hypercalcemia
- Creatinine clearance decreased by 30%
- Evidence of kidney stones or nephrocalcinosis
- 24-hour urine calcium excretion > 400 mg
- Decreased bone density: T-score below −2.0

Pts who decline surgery or have contraindications, medical management includes:
- Bisphosphonates   - Calcitonin   - Phosphate replacement

Secondary hyperparathyroidism caused by chronic renal failure
Vitamin D supplementation and calcium salts
Some pts require parathyroidectomy.

S **Has the pt had weakness, fatigue, dizziness, polyuria, or excessive thirst?**
These symptoms are associated with cortisol and aldosterone deficiency.

Has the pt had any other symptoms suggestive of adrenal insufficiency?
- Nausea or vomiting   - Abdominal pain   - Anorexia
- Diarrhea   - Weight loss   - Salt cravings

Has the pt noticed any changes in skin color?
Skin hyperpigmentation (classic in primary AI and absent in secondary AI) occurs at scars, areolae, and creases, such as in the palms and groin area.

When did these symptoms begin?
The duration of symptoms can be either acute or chronic.
- Acute symptoms suggest things like hemorrhage, thrombosis, or necrosis.
- Chronic symptoms suggest autoimmune, TB, or adrenoleukodystrophy.

Does the pt or anyone in the family have autoimmune problems such as thyroid disease, type 1 diabetes, vitiligo, or lupus?
Increases the probability that the pt has autoimmune AI.

If the pt is a woman, has she noticed any changes in menstruation?
Amenorrhea may suggest secondary AI.

Does the pt have any headaches or visual changes?
These are symptoms associated with other pituitary hormones:
- Polyuria, polydipsia (diabetes insipidus)
- Headaches, visual changes (space-occupying lesions)

Ask the pt about HIV risk factors
Look for a history of AIDS or risk factors for HIV. Pts with AIDS are at risk for AI, especially due to infections (TB, fungal).

Has the pt ever developed a leg clot?
Antiphospholipid syndrome is associated with AI as well as thrombosis.

What medicines does the pt use?
Any of the following medications pose a risk for AI:
- Warfarin therapy   - Long-term steroid   - Ketoconazole   - Phenytoin

Does the pt have cancer or a history of previous cancer?
Metastatic tumors (lung, breast, kidney) or lymphoma cause AI (adrenal cortex).

O **Review VS**
Sepsis, hemorrhage: fever, tachycardia, hypotension
Aldosterone deficiency: orthostatic hypotension

Perform a PE
Altered mental status is commonly seen.
Look for signs of pituitary involvement.
- Stunted growth (growth hormone)
- Delayed puberty or depression, weight gain (hypothyroid)
Also look for signs of AI and its associated diseases:
- Hyperpigmentation   - Vitiligo
- Thinning of axillary or pubic hair   - Thyroid enlargement

What are the results of CBC and chemistry panel?
Common abnormalities: normocytic anemia, low sodium, high potassium, elevated BUN/creatinine, low glucose

Perform diagnostic tests
Check cortisol, adrenocorticotropic hormone (ACTH)
- Primary AI = low cortisol, high ACTH (> 100 pg/mL)
- Secondary/Tertiary AI = low cortisol, low ACTH

Cosyntropin test = an ACTH stimulation to evaluate adrenal response:
Check AM cortisol, give 250 mcg cosyntropin IV, repeat cortisol after 60 minutes.
- Normal = post-stimulation cortisol at least 18 mcg/dL more than initial
- Primary AI = no increase in cortisol

If you suspect secondary AI, consider a metyrapone test, insulin-induced hypoglycemia.

Consider imaging studies
CXR to look for evidence of TB or lung mass
Head MRI to rule out pituitary tumor
Abdominal CT to look for enlarged adrenal glands or calcifications

Consider biopsy of adrenal mass for definitive diagnosis

Adrenal Insufficiency
Can be primary (adrenal) or secondary (central: CNS). Corticotropin-releasing factor is released from the hypothalamus, stimulating ACTH release from the pituitary, stimulating the adrenals to release cortisol. The adrenals also make aldosterone and androgens.

Primary AI causes include:		Secondary AI
- Autoimmune	- Lymphoma	- Pituitary tumors
- Tuberculosis	- Hemorrhage	- Craniopharyngioma
- AIDS	- Necrosis	- Long-term steroid use
- Fungal infections	- Thrombosis	- Postpartum (Sheehan)
- Metastatic tumor	- Adrenoleukodystrophy	- Head trauma

Tertiary AI: hypothalamic tumors

Differential diagnosis and possible comorbidities
Acute: dementia, liver failure, acute renal failure, septic shock, diabetic ketoacidosis
Chronic: delirium, chronic fatigue syndrome, depression, dark skin, acanthosis nigricans, paraneoplastic syndrome

Determine if the AI is acute or chronic
The dose of hydrocortisone depends on this.

If acute AI, initiate workup but do not wait for results, because this condition is life-threatening. Give hydrocortisone 100 mg bolus, then 100 to 200 mg IV over 24 hrs and fluid resuscitation with IV fluid
Without cortisol replacement (hydrocortisone), pt is less likely to respond appropriately to stressors (surgery, sepsis). One of the ways pts respond poorly is vasodilation, which can be addressed with both hydrocortisone and IV fluid.

If chronic AI, give hydrocortisone 20 to 30 mg/day
Chronic AI requires only replacement (< 30 mg) rather than stress dose (100 mg).

Determine if it is primary or secondary/tertiary chronic AI
If primary AI, give fludrocortisone (mineralocorticoid replacement) 0.05 to 1.0 mg/day.
Regardless of type of AI, workup underlying cause and treat

S **Does the pt complain of proximal muscle weakness?**
Pt may report difficulty in arising from a chair or climbing stairs.

Does the pt report weight gain?
Increased cortisol results in distributory weight gain.
- Moon facies   - Pendulous abdomen   - Cervical fat pad

Is there evidence of androgen excess?
- Hirsutism   - Oligomenorrhea/amenorrhea
- Acne   - Decreased libido

Does the pt have a history of conditions associated with cortisol excess?
- Hypertension   - Kidney stones   - Diabetes mellitus   - Osteoporosis

Review medications
Long-term glucocorticoids: Systemic is most common, but topical, inhaled, and intra-articular still pose some risk.

O **Examine the VS for signs of excess cortisol**
Hypertension

Perform a complete PE, looking especially for
Gen: central obesity, thin extremities
Skin: thin, dry, ecchymosis, violaceous stria of abdomen or proximal extremities, hirsute, acne, muscle wasting
HEENT: cataracts, moon facies, facial plethora, supraclavicular fullness, buffalo hump (cervical fat pad)
Abd: mass

Review basic metabolic panel
The K and Cl will tend to be low, whereas the bicarb and glucose will be high.

Perform a screening test
Overnight dexamethasone suppression test
- Administer 1 g dexamethasone at 11 PM, then measure cortisol at 8 AM.
- AM cortisol < 5 mcg/dL rules out Cushing's syndrome
Consider 24-hr urine collection for cortisol.
- Increased serum cortisol results in an increased filtered cortisol.
- Urine cortisol > 40 in a woman or > 80 μg/dL in a man suggests Cushing's syndrome.

Order tests needed to determine etiology
Distinguish between adrenocorticotropic hormone (ACTH)-dependent and ACTH-independent.
Check cortisol, ACTH between midnight and 2 AM. If the cortisol is high (> 15 μg/dL), look at the ACTH:
- ACTH (< 5 pg/mL) suggests adrenal tumor
- ACTH 5–24 pg/mL requires CRH stimulation test
- ACTH 25–150 pg/mL suggests Cushing's disease
- ACTH > 150 pg/mL (usually ~ 500) suggests ectopic production

Order appropriate imaging
Consider MRI sella turcica to rule out pituitary adenoma.
Consider MRI of adrenal glands to rule out adrenal tumors, and if it is positive for adrenal tumor, consider measuring 24-hr urine ketosteroids.
- > 30 mg/24 hr indicates carcinoma
- Low excretion indicates adenoma

Consider CT chest/abdomen/pelvis to rule out malignancy.

Consider petrosal venous sinus catheterization and measurement of ACTH

If above imaging is negative, measurement distinguishes pituitary versus ectopic ACTH.

Cushing's Syndrome

A condition characterized by round facies, cervical fat pad, purple abdominal striae, truncal obesity, and muscle wasting, caused by excess endogenous (from the adrenal cortex) or exogenous glucocorticoids

Cushing's Disease

The same as the syndrome except that the excess glucocorticoids are caused by excess ACTH from the pituitary. To quickly review, the hypothalamus makes cortisol-releasing hormone (CRH), which stimulates the release of ACTH from the pituitary. ACTH stimulates the release of glucocorticoids from the adrenal cortex.

Differential diagnosis

Pituitary adenoma
Ectopic CRH secretion
Adrenal tumors or hyperplasia
Long-term steroid therapy
Ectopic ACTH production

- Small cell lung carcinoma	- Bronchial carcinoids
- Pheochromocytoma	- Medullary thyroid carcinoma

Pseudo-Cushing's

- Obesity	- Chronic alcoholism
- Hypothyroidism	- Insulinoma

Monitor glucose and lipids closely and treat as indicated

Diabetes and hyperlipidemia are well-recognized effects of glucocorticoid excess.

Recognize and treat osteoporosis with calcium, vitamin D, and bisphosphonate therapy if necessary

Recognize that Cushing's places the pt at higher risk for osteoporosis.

Consider starting the pt on a proton pump inhibitor

Pts with Cushing's are also at higher risk of peptic ulcer disease.

Treat Cushing's disease (pituitary adenoma) with surgery, glucocorticoid replacement, and if necessary irradiation

Transsphenoidal resection of microadenoma is curative in more than 80% of pts.
Give replacement glucocorticoids daily for 6 to 12 months postoperatively.
If no cure after resection, therapy includes pituitary irradiation.
Few pts may need bilateral adrenalectomy for cure.

Treat ectopic ACTH- or CRH-producing tumors with surgery or medical management of symptoms

If possible, resect underlying tumor.

Treat high cortisol with adrenal enzyme inhibitors (ketoconazole or metyrapone)

Treat hypokalemia with spironolactone

Resect adrenal tumors surgically when possible and provide replacement glucocorticoids

Bilateral adrenalectomy (bilateral hyperplasia)
Unilateral adrenalectomy (unilateral adenoma or carcinoma)

S

Does the pt have risk factors for osteoporosis (OP)?
Any of the following pose a risk for OP:

- Thin (low body weight)
- Female
- Family history of fractures
- Elderly (Age > 65)
- Smoking
- Postmenopausal
- Caffeine intake
- Caucasian
- Previous fractures
- Alcohol
- Eating disorder (bulimia, anorexia nervosa)

Does the pt report bone pain?
A bone fracture may be the first presentation of underlying OP.

Does the pt report a loss of height?
Typically, the pt has 2 to 4 cm loss in height.

Does the pt have a history of prolonged immobilization?
Pts who are paralyzed or bedridden may suffer significant bone loss.

Does the pt have a history of endocrinopathy?
A pt with any of the following disorders is at risk for developing OP:

- Hyperthyroidism
- Cushing's syndrome
- Hyperparathyroidism
- Diabetes mellitus

Is there a family history of disorders associated with OP?

- Ehlers-Danlos syndrome
- Marfan syndrome
- Hemochromatosis

Review medications
Any of the following drugs pose a risk for OP:

- Chronic steroid therapy
- Phenytoin
- Benzodiazepines
- High doses of thyroid hormone
- Phenobarbital

O

Review VS and perform a PE
Measure height and weight and look at habitus.
Look for thyromegaly or thyroid mass.
Look at spine for kyphosis (anterior curvature of thoracic spine).
Palpate ribs for occult fractures, and perform full skeletal exam.

Review the results of the pt's CBC and comprehensive metabolic panel
There are no diagnostic lab abnormalities in OP.
Rarely, alkaline phosphatase and calcium may be increased.

Perform a dual-energy x-ray absorptiometry (DEXA) scan
Indications include:

- All women > age 60
- Hyperparathyroidism
- Long-term steroid therapy
- Postmenopausal women with risk factors
- Abnormal x-ray (osteopenia, fracture)

Diagnostic criteria:
- T-score < -2.5, OP
- T-score < -1.0, increased risk of OP

Pts with suspected secondary causes require further lab tests
Check TSH and, if abnormal, free T4.
Check PTH, increased in hyperparathyroidism, decreased in malignancy).
Check 24-hr urinary calcium excretion.
- Decreased (< 50 mg/24 hr) in malabsorption or malnutrition
- Increased (> 300 mg/24 hr) in high bone turnover states
Check fasting glucose.
Check free urine cortisol.

Consider spine x-ray
Especially in pt with documented height loss of 1 to 1.5 inches

Osteoporosis
Weakness of bone resulting from loss of bone mass, causing increased risk of fractures
There are three major types of primary osteoporosis:
- Type I: Usually occurs in > 50-year-old postmenopausal women
  - Lack of estrogen causes increased trabecular bone loss.
  - Associated with distal forearm and vertebral body fractures.
- Type II: Men and Women > 70 y/o
  - Increased loss of both cortical and trabecular bone loss.
  - Associated with fractures of pelvis; and proximal humerus, tibia, and neck.
- Idiopathic: Occurs in younger age groups; likely caused by unidentified secondary cause

Etiologies
- Idiopathic
- Malabsorption (Osteomalacia)
- Prolonged use of steroids
- Hyperparathyroidism
- Renal disease/failure
- Cushing's syndrome
- Disuse atrophy
- Menopause (without HRT)

Differential diagnosis
- Physical abuse
- Bone tumor
- Paget's disease
- Accidental trauma
- Advanced untreated thalassemia
- Secondary causes (see Etiologies)
- Multiple myeloma
- Osteogenesis imperfecta
- Metastases
- Leukemia/Lymphoma
- Osteomyelitis

Identify fractures and consult orthopedics for management
If pt has a hip or spinal fracture, evaluate for signs of internal blood loss or spinal cord compression. If noted, admit pt and make consultation emergent.

Obtain a pain score and address/control the pain
In mild cases, analgesics such as NSAIDs should be sufficient, but in cases involving fractures, such as those mentioned above, narcotics will likely be needed.
Calcitonin spray has also been found to be of benefit in some cases.

Educate all pts about how to prevent OP
The key to reducing OP is primary prevention. It is much more effective to prevent OP than to try to treat it when the pt has developed it.

Discuss simple changes the pt can make at home to avoid fractures
- Smoking cessation
- Medication adjustments
- Alcohol abstinence
- Weight-bearing exercises
- Home safety to prevent falls. Occupational Therapist can visit the home.

Give supplementation to improve bone strength
Calcium 1000–1200 mg per day
Vitamin D (200–600 IU per day)

Consider treatment with medical therapy
- Estrogens
- PTH
- Bisphosphonates (alendronate, risedronate)
- SERMS (raloxifene), or nasal calcitonin

S **Does the pt have risk factors for coronary artery disease (CAD)?**
Major risk factors include:
- Smoking   - Hypertension   - Diabetes
- Age (men > 45 years, women > 55 years)
- First-degree relative with early CAD (men < 55 years, women < 40 years)
Other risk factors (not considered major) include:
- Obesity   - Physical inactivity

Does the pt have CAD equivalents?
The following are considered equivalent to CAD:
- Peripheral artery disease   - Carotid artery stenosis
- Abdominal aortic aneurysm   - Diabetes mellitus (DM)

Does the pt have medical problems that secondarily cause dyslipidemia?
Any of the following disease states pose a risk for abnormal lipids:
- Hypothyroidism   - DM
- Chronic renal failure   - Long-term steroid use

O **Review VS and perform a PE**
Some findings to note are obesity, earlobe creases, thyromegaly, arcus senilis, and xanthomas.

What are the results of renal and liver function tests?
Increased BUN/Cr; if chronic suggest secondary cause
Abnormal LFTs: contraindication for lipid-lowering agents

Check lipid panel
All pts age 20 years and older should get a fasting lipid panel every 5 years.
According to ATP III classification:

Low-Density Lipoprotein

(LDL) cholesterol		Total cholesterol	
< 100	normal	< 200	desirable
101–129	near or > optimal	200–239	borderline
130–159	borderline high	> 240	high
160–190	high	> 190	very high

High-Density Lipoprotein

(HDL) cholesterol			
> 60	optimal	< 40	low

Look for the metabolic syndrome
Pts with any three of the following criteria have metabolic syndrome:
- Waist circumference > 40 inches in men, > 35 inches in women
- Fasting triglycerides > 150 mg/dL
- HDL cholesterol < 40 mg/dL in men, < 50 mg/dL in women
- Blood pressure > 130/85 mm Hg
- Fasting plasma glucose > 110 mg/dL

A **Dyslipidemia**
Abnormal lipoprotein levels: high cholesterol (> 200), triglycerides (> 150), LDLs (> 130), or low HDLs (< 40 in men, < 50 in women)

Etiology
Primary (genetic)
Secondary:

- Hypothyroidism   - Obstructive liver disease   - DM
- Long-term steroid use   - Chronic renal failure

P **Educate the pt about the risks of the disease and importance of lifestyle**

Lifestyle modifications such as exercise, nutrition (low-fat diet), and weight loss are the first-line treatment of dyslipidemias.

In order to be motivated to make such changes, the pt must understand the consequences (stroke, MI, peripheral vascular disease) of the disease.

Optimize treatment of any secondary causes
This not only improves the dyslipidemia but also addresses two problems or risk factors at once. If a diabetic has better glycemic control, it will be easier to control lipids, and both of those things are important improvements.

Count the number of risk factors to determine target goals of medical therapy
Pts with CAD or CAD equivalent (LDL goal < 100 mg/dL):

- LDL > 130 mg/dL: initiate drug therapy
- LDL 100–129 mg/dL:
  - Lifestyle modification for 3 months
  - Initiate drug therapy if no improvement after 3 months

Pts with more than two risk factors (LDL goal < 130 mg/dL):

- LDL > 130 mg/dL:
  - Initiate lifestyle modification for 3 months. Repeat lipid panel. In 6 weeks, if not improved, intensify lifestyle changes.
- Initiate drug therapy if > 130, after 3 months, and repeat lipid panel in 6 weeks.

Pts with zero to one risk factors (LDL goal < 160 mg/dL):

- Initiate lifestyle modification for 3 months. If persist 160–189 mg/dL, then begin drug therapy.

Treatment with lipid-lowering agents
Cholesterol-lowering drugs are listed in Table 9, with the more common, easily tolerated drugs at the top and the less used, lesser tolerated drugs at the bottom.

Table 9 Lipid-Lowering Agents			
Drugs	**Lower LDL**	**Lower TG**	**Increase HDL**
Statins	++	+	+
Fibric Acids	+	++	+
Nicotinic Acids	+	++	++
Bile Acid Resins	+	– –	–

IX

Rheumatology

S   **Is the pt over the age of 50, a smoker, experiencing weight loss, or have any history of cancer?**
A clinician's greatest concern is to rule out the worst possible diagnoses, in this case, vertebral metastases.

Is there a history of IV drug use or is the pt a diabetic?
Consider osteomyelitis in these pts.

Is there a history of recurrent urinary tract infections or kidney stones?
Pyelonephritis and renal colic can masquerade as low back pain.

Is there a history of gastroesophageal reflux?
If so, this may represent a perforated ulcer.

Does the pain radiate down the buttock and below the knee?
This is a common presentation of nerve root irritation. Etiologies include:
-      - Herniated disk   - Sciatica
-      - Spinal stenosis   - Sacroiliitis

How does rest affect the pain?
Most degenerative joint diseases of the back improve with rest and worsen with activity.
Pain that is unrelieved by rest or supine position and continues at night is worrisome for malignancy, infection, or cauda equina involvement.
Ankylosing spondylitis can actually improve with activity and worsen with rest.

Are there any symptoms of a cauda equina process?
-      - Multiple nerve root   - Bilateral leg weakness   - Incontinence
         involvement   - Rapidly evolving symptoms
-      - Decreased perineal sensation

O   **Conduct a neurologic exam of the back, hip, and lower extremities**
This will help rule out the more serious diagnoses. Observe for signs of multiple nerve root involvement because this suggests a cauda equina process (tumor, abscess).
Point tenderness over a vertebral body can suggest osteomyelitis or vertebral metastases.
Perform Schober's test:
- Begin by measuring 5 cm and 10 cm above the level of S1, first while standing up straight, and then again after bending forward with flexion at the hip.
- Normally there should be an increase of $\geq$ 5 cm between these two points with flexion.
- If the distance increases only 4 cm or less with flexion, consider ankylosing spondylitis or another one of the seronegative spondyloarthropathies.
Straight-leg test (pain radiating down the leg with less than 60 degrees of raising) suggests nerve root irritation in L4-L5 or L5-S1.
Decreased sensation over the medial calf, decreased dorsiflexion of the foot, and increased knee tendon jerk are suggestive of L4 nerve root involvement.
Decreased sensation over the medial aspect of the foot and decreased dorsiflexion of the great toe suggests L5 nerve root involvement.
Decreased sensation over the lateral aspect of the foot, decreased eversion of the foot, and increased ankle jerk suggests S1 nerve root involvement.

Look for any other nonrheumatologic causes of low back pain

Cachexia, breast mass, lymphadenopathy, urinary retention, and enlarged prostate are examples of signs of different malignancies.

Abdominal mass or bruit could signify the presence of an aneurysm.

Low Back Pain

The following five diagnoses are the most severe causes of back pain and should be ruled out with the initial exam when possible:

- Cancer: vertebral metastases, cauda equina tumor
- Infection: osteomyelitis, cauda equina abscess
- Fracture
- Ankylosing spondylitis
- Nonrheumatologic conditions: pancreatitis, aortic aneurysm, or perforated ulcer

If you suspect any of these diagnoses, an urgent and aggressive workup is required.

With these more serious diagnoses out of the way, the remaining diagnoses can be treated more conservatively:

| - Disk herniation | - Muscle strain | - Sciatica |
| - Sacroiliitis | - Degenerative joint disease | |

These are the most common causes of low back pain and any one of them can be extremely debilitating for the pt.

For pts in whom you suspect one of the first five diagnoses, order a plain radiograph of the lumbar spine immediately

If you do not suspect these diagnoses, proceed with conservative management for 2 to 4 weeks because most low back problems will resolve completely within this time.

If after 2 to 4 weeks symptoms still persist, you should order a plain film at that time.

Order an MRI urgently in any pt who displays cauda equina signs

If the MRI is positive, seek a neurosurgical consultation immediately.

Otherwise, institute conservative measures such as

Reassurance and education (how to properly lift): These are the foundations that the pt needs, particularly because the pain could take as long as 4 to 6 weeks to resolve.

Bed rest: Many pts want bed rest or feel that it is important. Bed rest should not be continued for more than 2 days.

Physical therapy: After a maximum of 2 days of bed rest, pts should engage in gentle back-mobilizing exercises.

Analgesia: Pain can usually be treated with NSAIDs. Reserve opioids for severe pain, and even then, for no more than 2 weeks.

Refer to orthopedic surgery if a documented herniation fails to respond to 6 weeks of conservative therapy for consideration of a lumbar discectomy.

S **Does the pt report any warmth, swelling, or acute pain at the joint?**
Rule out septic joint, because failure to do so may result in permanent disability.
Risk factors for septic joint include IV drug abuse and damaged joints.
Sexually active people (especially women during menses and pregnancy) are at risk for
  gonococcal infection.

How many joints are involved?
Monoarticular involves one joint (septic arthritis, Lyme disease).
Oligo- or pauciarticular involves 2 to 4 joints.
Polyarthritis involves more than 5 joints (SLE, RA).

When did the symptoms begin?
Acute duration is less than 6 weeks.
Chronic is more than 6 weeks.
The following viruses can cause polyarthritis that subsides in 6 weeks:
          - Rubella   - Mumps   - Human parvovirus B19   - Enterovirus

What joints are involved?
Rheumatoid arthritis (RA): metacarpophalangeal, PIP, wrists, and MTP
Osteoarthritis (OA): DIP, PIP, and carpometacarpal, weight-bearing joints
Gout: 1st MTP

Does pt report any morning stiffness?
Helps distinguish inflammatory (RA) from noninflammatory (OA) arthropathy.
Morning stiffness (> 1 hr in RA, < 1 hr in OA) is an inflammatory symptom.
Swelling, tenderness, warmth, and fever are also inflammatory symptoms.

Is the pain precipitated by motion or weight bearing and relieved with rest?
These are noninflammatory symptoms associated with OA rather than RA.

Does the pt report fever, chills, or malaise?
If so, consider septic arthritis, SLE, gout, or RA.

Focus the review of systems on a systemic rheumatologic disease
          - Alopecia   - Oral ulcers - Dysphagia   - Rash   - Hematuria
          - Dry mouth/eyes - Myopathy   - Photosensitivity - Raynaud's

O **Review VS for signs of systemic illness**
Fever indicates inflammatory arthritis.
Hypotension suggests septic shock from septic joint: address emergently.

Perform a PE
This will give information about joint pain and disability.
Gen: Assess ability to bear weight (wheelchair bound or use of canes, crutches).
HEENT: uveitis, conjunctivitis, episcleritis
Joint: Feel for warmth, soft tissue edema, and tenderness; test for range of motion.
Skin: urticaria, purpura, psoriasis, subcutaneous nodules, tophi, Heberden's (DIP) and
  Bouchard's (PIP) nodes.

Perform an arthrocentesis for an effusion, and review the results
Can help exclude or differentiate between:
          - Septic joint   - Gout   - CPDD
Contraindications to arthrocentesis include:
          - Cellulitis   - Bleeding disorders   - Uncooperative pt

Check gross appearance, cell count with differential, Gram stain, culture, crystals.
- Noninflammatory: < 3,000/μL WBC, < 25% PMN
- Inflammatory: > 3,000/μL WBC, > 50% PMN
- Purulent: > 50,000/μL WBC, > 90% PMN
- Gout: negatively birefringent crystals
- CPDD: weakly positive birefringent crystals

Review CBC
Leukocytosis, especially with left shift indicative of infection

Review the results of renal and liver function tests and urinalysis
Renal and liver involvement are common with rheumatologic disease.

Check ESR and CRP (nonspecific markers of inflammation)
CRP is a more reliable marker of acute phase response than ESR.

Consider further serologic tests
Consider antinuclear antibody if suspect rheumatologic disease.
Check rheumatoid factor, if suspect RA.
- A negative test does not rule out RA, 30% with seronegative RA.
- High titers are more diagnostic and indicate poor prognosis.

Polyarthritis
Inflammation of multiple joints at once

Etiologies
Noninflammatory: OA, trauma
Inflammatory:

- RA	- Gout	- Pseudogout
- SLE	- Scleroderma	- Fungal
- TB	- Reactive arthritis	- Juvenile rheumatoid arthritis

Purulent: Bacterial

Differential diagnosis

- Arthrogryposis	- Osteomalacia	- Crohn's disease
- Renal osteodystrophy	- Hemarthrosis	- Vaso-occlusive disease
- Tendonitis	- Fibromyalgia	

Identify septic joint and consult orthopedic surgeon for drainage
Failure to identify septic joint will result in permanent damage.

Panculture and start broad-spectrum antibiotics
Most common organisms are *S. aureus*, strep, gram negative.
If suspect gonococcal arthritis, start ceftriaxone 1 g IV qd.
Lyme (*B burgdorferi*): doxycycline 100 mg bid or amoxicillin 500 mg tid for 3 to 4 weeks
TB: four anti-TB meds (e.g., INH, rifampin, PZA, and ethambutol)
Candida: fluconazole 200 mg bid

Identify OA and begin treatment with lifestyle changes and anti-inflammatory medications
Weight loss and physical therapy
NSAIDs, glucosamine, capsaicin cream

Gout and pseudogout (See Crystal-Induced Arthropathy, p. 151)
RA (See RA, p. 152)
SLE (See SLE, p. 158)
Scleroderma (See Systemic Sclerosis, p. 162)

S **What is the pt's age?**
Acute gout is common in men age 30 to 60 years.
In women, gout usually occurs after menopause.
Early age onset (< 25 years) suggests a genetic component.

Does the pt report a history of alcohol and/or high-protein foods?
High-protein foods and some alcohols, worsen gout by increasing uric acid load.
Alcohol can also worsen gout by inhibiting enzymatic clearance of uric acid.

Is there a family history of arthropathy predisposing disorders?
Lesch-Nyhan syndrome, X-linked
Calcium pyrophosphate deposition disease (CPDD), AD
Polycystic kidney disease
- Glycogen storage disease, AR - Sickle cell   - Leukemia
- Medullary cystic kidney   - B-thalassemia

How long have symptoms been present?
Acute duration is typically defined by days to a few weeks.

What specific joints are involved?
Gout is commonly monoarticular, metatarsophalangeal of great toe, but also frequently
  in ankle.
CPDD involves knee most commonly, but can be seen in all joints.

Does the pt report any precipitating factors?
- Recent trauma or illness   - Postop   - Alcohol use

Review medications, especially those known to increase uric acid level
- Thiazide or loop diuretics   - Nicotinic acid
- Cyclophosphamide (post-transplant)   - Pyrazinamide

Does the pt have a history of kidney stones?
May precede symptoms of gout.

 Review the VS
Due to inflammation in gout and CPDD, fever may be present.
Hypertension and obesity are commonly associated with gout.

Perform PE, paying particular attention to the following
Joints: Feel for warmth, tenderness, effusions, and look for erythema.
Ext: Valgus knees suggest CPDD
Skin: tophi (urate crystal deposit), especially on ears

What are the results of the arthrocentesis?
Both CPDD and gout reveal inflammatory fluids.
Send cell count, Gram stain, and cultures because septic arthritis is common.
Look carefully for crystals.
- Gout (monosodium urate): needle shaped, (−) birefringence.
- CPDD: rhomboid, weakly (+).

**What are the results of the CBC, ESR, and comprehensive
metabolic panel?**
There are no diagnostic abnormalities common to gout or CPDD.
- Leukocytosis and increased ESR is caused by inflammation.
- Increased BUN and creatinine may suggest urate-induced nephropathy.

Consider uric acid level
This is not diagnostic and may be normal even in acute gout attack.
The risk of developing kidney stones is more than 50% if levels are > 13 mg/dL.

Consider the following lab tests if suspect CPDD-associated disorders
- Hypothyroidism (TSH)   - Hemochromatosis (ferritin)
- Hyperparathyroidism (calcium, PTH)   - Amyloidosis (fat biopsy)

Consider x-ray, looking for characteristic findings
CPDD: punctate or linear densities (chondrocalcinosis) in articular cartilage
Gout: varies, may see soft tissue swelling or in chronic stages can see atrophic or
   hypertrophic erosions (overhanging edge)

Consider 24-hr urine collection for uric acid to differentiate overproducers from underexcreters in gout
More than 800 mg/24 hr suggests overproduction.

Crystal-induced arthropathy
Joint inflammation related to overproduction and subsequent crystallization of a
   molecule such as monosodium urate in the case of gout or CPDD in pseudogout.

Differential diagnosis
- Septic joint   - Gout   - Pseudogout
- Osteoarthritis   - Rheumatoid arthritis   - Adult-onset stills
- Cellulitis   - Reactive arthritis   - Psoriatic arthritis

P

Rule out septic joint in acute monoarticular arthropathy by aspirating the joint
Send fluid for both Gram stain and crystals.
If suspicious for septic joint, treat empirically with broad-spectrum antibiotics until
   results of tap are obtained.

Treat acute gout/CPDD with Indomethacin 50 mg po q 8 hours until symptoms resolve
Treatment is aimed at relieving symptoms of arthritis and decreasing inflammation.
Consider also giving colchicine 0.5 to 0.6 mg po qh until pain relief (max 8 mg/day and
   adjust dose for renal or liver disease).

If NSAIDs or colchicine are contraindicated, may use steroids
Either systemic or intraarticular steroids may be used.
Transplant pts can be treated with intra-articular steroids.

Do not use allopurinol because this may worsen attack
Allopurinol should not be started for at least 2 weeks after the acute attack.

Educate pts about prevention of gouty attacks
- Weight loss   - Avoid alcohol   - Low-purine diet   - Avoid aspirin

After acute attack, check 24-hour urine and serum uric acid to determine if pts are overproducers or underexcretors
Use allopurinol if pts are overproducers to decrease production or in pts with tophi,
   nephrolithiasis, and chronic renal insufficiency.
Although some pts are underexcretors of uric acid, these pts should still be treated with
   allopurinol.
   • This is because uricosuric agents, such as probenecid, require that the pt take in
     greater than 1500 mL/day of water and have a creatinine clearance of > 60 mL/
     min. Pts may be unable to meet these expectations.

S How long have the symptoms been present?

Generally, RA is a chronic disease (symptoms present for more than 6 weeks).
If acute (less than 6 weeks), consider infectious or crystal-induced etiologies.

Does the pt report morning stiffness?

With RA, pts complain of morning stiffness lasting at least 1 hour.
With OA, morning stiffness lasts less less than 30 minutes.

What joints are involved?

MTPs may be the first joints involved.
Wrists, MCPs, PIPs, TMJ, and knees are commonly involved.
DIPs, lumbar spine, and SI joints are generally spared in RA.

How many joints are involved?

RA is generally considered polyarticular and symmetrical.

Does the pt report any systemic symptoms?

- Fever   - Chills   - Weight loss   - Fatigue   - Anorexia

Does the pt report extra-articular manifestations associated with RA?

Dry eyes, dry mouth (Sjögren's syndrome)
Dysphagia or dysphonia (inflammation of cricoarytenoid joint)
Acute paresthesias (mononeuritis multiplex)
Chest pain, shortness of breath, change in exercise tolerance (pleuritis)

O Review VS

Fever may be present from inflammation or underlying infection.

Perform a PE

Gen: Assess the pt's functional capacity.
HEENT: neck stiffness
- C1-2 subluxation increases risk of spinal cord compression.
- Requires further assessment with lateral flexion cervical spine x-rays.

Abd: splenomegaly
- Recall triad RA, splenomegaly, and neutropenia in Felty's syndrome.

Joint:
- Feel for warmth, tenderness, effusions, and synovial thickening.
- Look for erythema, edema, and test for range of motion.
- Look for deformities:
  - Flexion contracture
  - Ulnar deviation at MCP
  - Swan-neck deformities (flexion DIP, hyperextension PIP)
  - Boutonniere deformity (flexion PIP, hyperextension DIP)

Skin: Look for nodules over pressure points like extensor surfaces of upper extremities.
Neuro: Perform Phalen's and Tinel's tests. (Carpal tunnel syndrome is common in RA.)

Review the result of arthrocentesis if palpable effusion is present

Inflammatory fluid common with WBC > 20,000 (mostly PMNs), without crystals

Consider x-rays

Early in disease, x-rays are normal.
Erosions are not present until months or years after disease onset.

Review the results of the CBC, liver, and renal function tests

Obtain baseline values; some medications used to treat RA may be contraindicated.

Check the pt's rheumatoid factor (RF)
RF positive found in 85% of pts with RA.

RF titer correlates with severity; higher values denote worse prognosis, but it is not necessary to follow titer once documented to be positive.

RF can also be positive in chronic infectious/inflammatory states (systemic lupus erythematosus [SLE], tuberculosis, carcinoma).

Consider erythrocyte sedimentation rate (ESR)
This is a nonspecific inflammatory marker for following the course of disease.

Consider CXR
Findings include interstitial fibrosis, lung nodules (Caplan's syndrome-interstitial pneumoconiosis + nodules), pleurisy, and pleural effusions.

Thoracentesis generally reveals very low glucose levels, high lactate dehydrogenase.

Consider ECG
Findings include pericarditis and conduction abnormalities.

Echocardiogram may reveal valvular abnormalities.

A **Rheumatoid Arthritis**
Autoimmune inflammation of the articular cartilage of multiple joints for longer than 6 months. Diagnose if at least 4 of the 7 following criteria are met:
1. Morning stiffness (at least 1 hour) for 6 weeks
2. Swelling of hand joints (wrists, MCP, PIP) for 6 weeks
3. Swelling of three or more joints
4. Symmetric joint swelling for 6 weeks
5. Rheumatoid nodules
6. Erosive synovitis on x-ray of the hands
7. RF positive

Differential diagnosis
- Osteoarthritis   - Gout/Pseudogout   - SLE
- Scleroderma   - Juvenile rheumatoid   - Spondyloarthropaties
- Rheumatic fever   arthritis   - Polymyalgia rheumatica

P **Diagnosis of rheumatoid arthritis is life changing; discuss disease progression, treatment options, side effects, and prognosis**
Pt education is crucial for adherence to therapy and subsequent disease control.

Refer to rheumatologist and physical therapy early in disease
Experience/expertise in RA management makes a significant difference.

Occupational and physical therapy are important for maintenance and preservation of function as the disease progresses.

Treat joint pain and swelling with NSAIDs or COX-2 inhibitors
This will help address the pain and discomfort of the disease.

Use disease-modifying antirheumatic drugs to limit joint damage
Hydroxychloroquine: regular ophthalmology follow-up (retinopathy)

Sulfasalazine: monitor CBC

Methotrexate: monitor CBC, LFT, renal function, folate supplementation

Tumor necrosis factor inhibitors: Remicade, Enbrel

Low-dose glucocorticoids

Treat refractory extra-articular manifestations with systemic steroids
Steroids will not modify the disease, but they can make the pt feel better.

Surgical referral for joint replacement or carpal tunnel release

S **What is the pt's age, racial background, and gender?**
There are associations between type of arthropathy and age, race, and gender:
- Ankylosing spondylitis (AS)
  - Presents in late twenties
  - M:F 5:1
  - Native Americans > other
- Reactive arthritis (Reiter's)
  - Young men
  - M:F 9:1
  - White > Black

Does the pt have a history of inflammatory bowel disease (IBD)?
Pts with IBD (Crohn's > ulcerative colitis) are at risk for arthritis.

Does the pt have a history of psoriasis, skin disease, or chronic rash?
Pts with psoriasis are at risk for psoriatic arthritis.

Does the pt report recent illness?
There are various illnesses associated with reactive arthritis:
- Occurs 2 to 4 weeks after infectious diarrhea: salmonella, shigella, campylobacter, clostridium, yersinia
- Genitourinary infections: chlamydia, ureaplasma
- Respiratory infections: *Chlamydia pneumoniae*

Does the pt report genitourinary symptoms?
Reactive syndrome includes urethritis:
- Dysuria   - Penile or vaginal discharge

Does the pt have eye symptoms?
Reactive arthritis includes conjunctivitis:
- Eye pain   - Redness   - Eyelid crusting
AS associated with uveitis:
- Unilateral pain   - Photophobia   - Lacrimation

Ask specifically about joint pain
Asymmetrical oligoarticular pain
LE joint involvement typical for reactive arthritis.
Hand distal interphalangeal (DIP) joints suggests psoriatic arthritis.
Back pain, if worse with rest and improved with exercise, is typical for AS.
Buttock pain that radiates into the thigh, worse with rest, suggests sacroiliitis.

O **Review VS and perform a PE**
Skin: rash on palms or soles
- Keratoderma blennorrhagicum associated with reactive arthritis.
- Psoriatic arthritis: pitting nails, scaly lesions on elbow, knees
Ext: dactylitis (sausage digits)
Eye: conjunctivitis (reactive arthritis), uveitis (AS)
Heart: listen for murmur (AI suggests aortitis in AS)
Genital: lesions on shaft of penis (circinata balanitis), cervical ulcer
Joint:
- Feel for warmth, tenderness, and edema; test for range of motion.
- Tenderness at tendon sites (enthesitis)
- Press on sacrum while pt is prone (sacroiliitis)

Check urinalysis
A pt suspected of having reactive arthritis must be ruled out for urethritis.
- Sterile pyuria suggests underlying venereal infection.
- Send *Chlamydia* antigen.

Send urethral and cervical cultures for *Chlamydia* and *N. gonorrhea*.

Review the result of arthrocentesis
Pt's synovial fluid most consistent with inflammatory process.
- Send Gram stain, bacterial, and *N. gonococcal* cultures.

Consider x-rays
Order x-rays of the feet for pts with heel pain: May have erosions of calcaneus.
Check a spinal x-ray on pts with AS: bamboo spine and fusion sacroiliac joint

Consider test for HLA-B27
The incidence of HLA-B27 is common, highest with AS more than 90%.

Seronegative Spondyloarthropathy
The seronegative spondyloarthropathies are a rather heterogeneous group of rheumatoid factor-negative conditions involving inflammation of the intervertebral joints.

Etiologies
- AS	- Psoriatic arthritis
- Reactive arthritis (Reiter's)	- IBD associated

Identify and treat septic arthritis
Acute monoarticular arthropathy must be ruled out for septic joint.
Treat pt empirically with broad-spectrum antibiotics until tap results are obtained

Treat AS with conservative measures and pain relief
Physical therapy for proper posture
Regular stretching and spinal exercise
NSAIDs (indomethacin or diclofenac)

Treat reactive arthritis by addressing uveitis, urethritis, and arthritis
If culture is positive for chlamydia, give azithromycin 1 g po one time
An alternative is doxycycline 100 mg po bid for 7 days.
Remember to also treat the partner.

Treat arthritis with NSAIDs (indomethacin or diclofenac)
Use COX-2 inhibitors if pt does not tolerate NSAIDs.
Use methotrexate or sulfasalazine in refractory cases.

For psoriatic arthritis, treat the psoriasis and address arthritis
Treatment arthritis with NSAIDs (indomethacin) as above, but may also use methotrexate or gold for refractory cases.
Do not use hydroxychloroquine or β-blockers because they can exacerbate skin disease.

Treat IBD-associated arthritis by addressing underlying disease; this is vital because arthritis is related to flares of IBD

S **What is the pt's age?**
Generally, myositis has a bimodal age distribution: 10–15 years and 50–60 years of age.
Malignancy-associated myositis and inclusion body myositis (IBM) are common
> 50 years.

What is the pt's racial background and gender?
African-Americans are affected more than Caucasians.
Women affected more than men (2:1), except with IBM men affected more than
women.

Ask about muscle pain
Onset is generally insidious.
Affects symmetrical proximal muscles (neck and proximal extremities).
  • Pt typically reports difficulty in rising from a chair or washing hair.
IBM is generally asymmetric, with distal muscle weakness.
Facial and ocular muscles are spared.
Dysphagia (especially with initiating swallowing) and dysphonia

Review medications
Many medications cause proximal muscle weakness:
  - Steroids   - Alcohol   - Statins
  - Colchicine   - Antiretrovirals

O **Review the pt's VS and perform a PE**
Skin: heliotrope rash, Gottron's papules, shawl sign (erythema shoulders and neck),
  V sign (chest, neck), mechanic hands
Lung: dry late inspiratory crackles (interstitial fibrosis)

Review CBC, liver, and renal function tests
Myopathies are often associated with occult malignancy.

Look for serologic markers of muscle damage
With myositis, muscle enzymes like CK, aldolase, AST, ALT, LDH should be elevated.

Consider checking antibodies to try to further delineate the type of myositis
Anti-Jo-1 Ab presents polymyositis more than dermatomyositis.
  • Associated with interstitial lung disease (ILD).
  • Associated with antisynthetase syndrome: myopathy, ILD, arthritis, Raynaud's
    phenomena, and mechanic hands.
Anti-Mi-2 is specific for dermatomyositis.
Anti-SRP (signal recognition particle) implies a poor prognosis.
  • Associated with cardiomyopathy and distal muscle involvement.

Consider EMG
This is not a diagnostic test because some pts have normal EMGs, but common
  findings include fibrillations, high-frequency discharge, and low amplitude.

Get a CXR
This may be normal, but look for signs of fibrosis.

Get a muscle biopsy
Necrosis and inflammation are seen with polymyositis and dermatomyositis.
Intracellular vacuoles and myeloid bodies are seen with IBM.

Chronic Inflammatory Myopathy

A group of idiopathic disorders in which muscle damage is caused by immune system activity (inflammation)

Etiologies

Polymyositis: proximal muscle weakness, elevated muscle enzymes, characteristic EMG

Dermatomyositis: proximal muscle weakness, heliotrope rash, Gottron's papules

Inclusion body myositis: proximal and distal muscle weakness, elevated muscle enzymes, usually over age 50 years old

Differential diagnosis

- Myositis associated with malignancy
- Thyroid disease
- Fibromyalgia
- Lupus (SLE)
- Muscular dystrophy
- Guillain-Barré syndrome
- Eaton-Lambert syndrome
- Myasthenia gravis
- Botulism
- Tick paralysis
- Drug-induced myopathy
- Sarcoid/HIV (associated with polymyositis)

Identify potential life-threatening complications, such as acute respiratory failure caused by respiratory muscle weakness, and admit pt to a monitored bed if indicated

Obtain ABG, if evidence of CO_2 retention, and monitor closely and prepare for intubation.

Screen for underlying malignancy

Dermatomyositis is associated with an increased risk for malignancy.

Educate pt about disease and prognosis

As with any disease, compliance is improved with good pt education.

Refer to physical or occupational therapy

To help with recovery as well as adaptations to muscle weakness

Obtain a swallow evaluation

To monitor for esophogeal dysfunction caused by polymyositis

Treat inflammatory myopathies with medications to reduce inflammation

Steroids (prednisone 40–60 mg qd)

Methotrexate or azathioprine can be used if the pt does not respond to steroids.

Monitor disease activity by changes in serum muscle enzymes

See above.

S **What is the pt's racial background and gender?**
Women, especially in their reproductive years, are affected more than men (9:1).
African-Americans and Hispanics are at increased risk.

Does the pt have a family history of systemic lupus erythematosus (SLE)?
High frequency is seen among first-degree relatives.
Commonly associated with HLA-DR2, HLA-DR3

Does the pt have coexisting autoimmune diseases?
Previous/current autoimmune disease is higher risk for another.
- Autoimmune thyroiditis   - Autoimmune hemolytic anemia
- ITP   - Sjögren's syndrome

Has the pt had recurrent spontaneous abortions or thrombosis?
There is an association between antiphospholipid syndrome and SLE.

Review medications for those associated with a lupus-like syndrome
- Procainamide   - Quinidine   - INH   - Hydralazine

Does the pt have any constitutional symptoms common in SLE?
- Fever   - Malaise   - Weight loss

Is there evidence that multiple organ systems are involved?
Mucocutaneous:
- Alopecia (patchy)   - Rash (malar or discoid)   - Oral ulcers
- Photosensitivity   - Dry eyes/mouth (Sjögren's syndrome)
Joints: Symmetric polyarticular distribution (proximal interphalangeal, metacarpophalangeal, wrists, knees) as in rheumatoid arthritis.
- Pain   - Stiffness   - Swelling
Pulmonary: hemoptysis, pleuritic chest pain, shortness of breath
Cardiac: pleuritic chest pain that changes with position (pericarditis)
CNS: mood changes, anxiety, memory loss, headache, change in vision
Raynaud's phenomena: changes in skin on exposure to cold or stress

O **Review the VS**
Fever is common and may indicate an underlying infection or active disease.
High blood pressure suggests underlying renal disease.
Hypotension (with distant heart sounds and jugular venous distention) indicates cardiac tamponade.

Perform a PE
Skin:
- Discoid (raised patch with overlying scale on face, scalp, ears, neck)
  - Alopecia   - Malar rash (spares nasolabial folds)   - Palpable purpura
HEENT: oral ulcers
Joint: Look for erythema; feel for warmth, edema, effusions, tenderness.
Heart: Listen for murmurs, pericardial friction rub.
Lung: decreased air entry; decreased tactile fremitus

Review CBC
- Leukopenia   - Anemia   - Thrombocytopenia

Check urinalysis
The presence of proteinuria and RBC casts suggest lupus nephritis.
- Consider 24-hour urine collection for protein and creatinine.
- Consider a renal ultrasound to assess kidney size.
- Renal biopsy is indicated if it will change the management course.

Check an antinuclear antibody (ANA)
Found in up to 95% of pts with SLE, but poor specificity.

Check anti-dsDNA and anti-Smith
Unique to SLE (100% specific, low sensitivity)
Anti-dsDNA is important for following renal involvement.

Check anti-Ro/La
Anti-Ro has a strong association with neonatal lupus and subacute cutaneous lupus.
Approximately 10% to 30% of mothers with anti-Ro will deliver babies with congenital heart block.

Check complement levels and erythrocyte sedimentation rate
Serologic markers for disease activity and inflammation

Systemic Lupus Erythematosus

Diagnosis requires 4 of the following 11 criteria:

1. Malar rash	7. Renal disorder (proteinuria, cellular casts)
2. Discoid rash	8. Immunologic markers (anti-dsDNA,
3. Neuro (Sz, Psychosis)	anti-Sm, or antiphospholipid Ab)
4. Oral ulcers	9. Serositis (pleuritis or pericarditis)
5. Photosensitivity	10. Heme (anemia/leukopenia/
6. Arthritis (> 2 joints)	thrombocytopenia)
	11. ANA (+)

A brief mnemonic is "MD NO PARISH ANA."

Differential diagnosis
Vasculitis: polyarteritis nodosa, microscopic polyangiitis, Wegener's granulomatosis
Infectious: HIV, syphilis, Epstein-Barr virus, brucellosis, Lyme disease
Rheumatic: rheumatoid arthritis, mixed connective tissue disease, Crohn's
Neoplasm: perineoplastic syndrome, leukemia, lymphoma

Identify any life-threatening illness in an SLE pt
CV: myocardial infarction, cardiac tamponade, pulmonary embolism, serositis
CNS: vasculitis, stroke
Infectious: subacute bacterial endocarditis, bacteremia, myocarditis, pericarditis, meningitis, septic arthritis
Rheumatologic: thrombotic thrombocytopenic purpura, ITP

Identify and remove precipitating factors such as medications (see above) that cause lupus-like syndrome
Removal of some medicines, like quinidine, result in resolution of the symptoms.

Treat coexisting autoimmune disorders
Remember that these pts are at increased risk for multiple autoimmune disorders, so pay attention to signs of other problems in the pt.

Treat SLE with anti-inflammatory/immunosuppressive agents
- NSAIDs, COX-2 inhibitors   - Steroids (oral, topical or intra-articular)
- Hydroxychloroquine   - Azathioprine
- Cyclophosphamide   - Methotrexate

S **Does the pt complain of malaise, fever, weight loss, or night sweats?**
Vasculitis commonly presents with nonspecific complaints such as these.

Does the pt complain of headaches or changes in vision?
If so, consider giant cell arteritis (GCA), especially in pts older than 60 with:
 - Throbbing pain   - Painless loss of vision (amaurosis fugax)

Does the pt report GI symptoms?
GCA: dysphagia, trismus, jaw claudication with chewing
Polyarteritis nodosa (PAN), microscopic polyangiitis (MPA), Henoch-Schönlein
  purpura (HSP): periumbilical pain, especially after eating, classical for mesenteric
  ischemia
PAN: cholecystitis and appendicitis
HSP: nausea/vomiting
PAN/HSP: GI blood loss

Does the pt report pulmonary symptoms?
Wegener/MPA/HSP: hemoptysis may be seen with pulmonary capillaritis
Wegener: recurrent sinus, ear, or upper respiratory infections
Churg-Strauss: asthma or allergic rhinitis

Does the pt report skin changes?
HSP: palpable purpura involving buttocks and lower extremities
Cryoglobulinemia: recurrent palpable purpura of lower extremities

Does the pt report joint or muscle pain?
HSP: arthritis of knees and ankles
Polymyalgia rheumatica (PMR): symmetric pain/stiffness in the hips/shoulders
PAN: myalgias involving calves

Ask the pt about neuropathy
PAN: mononeuritis multiplex

Ask about risk factors for hepatitis B or C
Up to 30% of PAN is associated with hepatitis B or C.
Cryoglobulinemia is common with hepatitis C.

O **Review VS**
          - Fever   - Hypertension (renin-mediated in PAN)

Perform a PE
HEENT: tender or nodular temporal artery, scalp tenderness (GCA); nasal mucosal
  lesions or saddle nose deformity (Wegener)
Neuro: foot drop (PAN, MPA)
Skin: livedo reticularis, ulcers (PAN), palpable purpura (MPA, HSP, cryoglobulinemia)

Check CBC
Eosinophilia (PAN, Churg-Strauss)

Check renal and liver function tests
Check erythrocyte sedimentation rate (ESR)
Check U/A
Look for hematuria, RBC casts, proteinuria (PAN, MPA, HSP).

Check ANCA
Order a CXR
Perform a renal biopsy

Vasculitis
Inflammation of blood vessels, usually causing multisystem disease
- Large vessel (> 150 μm)
  - Giant cell/temporal arteritis (GCA): Inflammation of the large arteries of the head and neck can lead to blindness.
  - Polymyalgia rheumatica (PMR): hip/shoulder stiffness
  - Takayasu arteritis (pulseless disease): inflammation of the aortic arch leading to arm claudication, amaurosis fugax, headache
- Medium vessel (diameter 50–150 μm)
  - Polyarteritis nodosa (PAN): Involves nearly all tissues but the lungs for an extremely variable presentation.
  - Buerger disease: Thrombophlebitis and eventually ischemia in the distal extremities. Exacerbated by smoking. Rarely involves internal organs.
- Small vessel (< 50 μm)
  - Henoch-Schönlein purpura (HSP): lower extremity palpable purpura, abdominal pain, and variable kidney involvement. Due to deposition of IgA.
  - Cryoglobulinemia: recurrent palpable purpura with darkening of skin on resolution of lesions. Associated with hepatitis C.
  - Wegener: Involves the respiratory tract and kidneys, leading to nosebleeds and renal failure. Associated with C-ANCA.
  - Microscopic polyangiitis (MPA): causes a pulmonary-renal presentation similar to Wegener's and Goodpasture's syndromes, P-ANCA
  - Churg-Strauss: asthma, eosinophilia, and P-ANCA

Differential diagnosis
If a pt presents with complaints from multiple organ systems, consider vasculitis along with the other great imitators.
Infectious: HIV, syphilis, Epstein-Barr virus
Neoplastic: perineoplastic syndromes
Autoimmune: systemic lupus erythematosus, mixed connective tissue disorder, Crohn's disease, celiac disease

P **Identify life-threatening complications of vasculitis and treat appropriately**
- Ischemic bowel or perforation
- Capillaritis or glomerulonephritis
- Sepsis/infections
- Thrombosis

Verify diagnosis with blood tests and biopsy if necessary. Consider consulting Rheumatology for more direction
Takayasu and GCA can be treated with steroids
Treat vision loss immediately with high-dose steroids to prevent blindness.
Treat stable pts with oral steroids.

Treat PMR with NSAIDs or low-dose steroids
Treat PAN with high-dose steroids
Use bactrim for PCP prophylaxis.

HSP is generally self-limited, but symptoms can be treated with NSAIDs for arthralgias
Cryoglobulinemia can be treated with INF alpha +/−ribavirin
Wegener's can be treated with high-dose steroids and cyclophosphamide
MPA can be treated with cyclophosphamide and steroids
Churg-Strauss can be treated with steroids

S **What is the pt's racial background and gender?**
The following groups are at risk for systemic sclerosis (SS):
- Females are affected more often than men (7:1).
- Native Americans are at highest risk.

Does the pt report environmental exposures?
There is a questionable association with some environmental toxins:
          - Silica dust   - Organic solvents
Secondary scleroderma is reported with:
          - Bleomycin   - Benzene   - Vinyl chloride

Does the pt have pruritus?
Pruritus can be the initial manifestation seen with skin involvement and is self-limited.

Does the pt have other organ system involvement?
Skin changes: thickening or tightness

Pulmonary symptoms: shortness of breath, dyspnea on exertion, cough
- Pts with SS are at risk for interstitial fibrosis and pulmonary hypertension.
- This is the number-one cause of mortality!

Cardiac symptoms: chest pain, palpitations
GI symptoms: dysphagia, malabsorption, constipation
Raynaud's phenomenon: changes in skin color on exposure to cold or stress
Musculoskeletal: arthralgias, myalgias

O **Review VS**
Accelerated hypertension suggests renal crisis (see below).

Perform a PE
Skin:
          - Telangiectasia (face, hands, mouth)   - Small mouth (tight, pursed lip)
          - Subcutaneous calcinosis   - Sclerodactyly
          - Nailfold capillaries, digital ulceration   - Hyper/hypopigmentation
Heart: jugular venous distention, loud P2; parasternal heave (pulmonary hypertension)
Joint: warmth, edema, tenderness; listen for tendon friction rubs.

Consider checking antinuclear antibody, anti-centromere, anti-SCL-70
There are no antibodies found in every pt with SS.
- Anticentromere antibody is found in 80% of CREST.
- Anti-SCL-70 (antitopoisomerase) is found in 20% of SS.

Consider CXR and hand x-rays
There is a risk of developing pulmonary disease, so check a baseline CXR.
Common abnormalities on hand films include:
- Joint calcinosis or osteolysis of fingertips

Consider an ECG
Pts are at risk for conduction abnormalities.

Consider pulmonary function tests
Pts typically have:
          - Restrictive lung pattern   - Decreased DLCO   - Lung volumes

Consider an echocardiogram
Pts are at risk for:
- Pulmonary hypertension   - Increased pulmonary artery pressure
- Diastolic dysfunction   > 35 mm Hg

Systemic Sclerosis
A connective tissue disease characterized by thickening and fibrosis of the skin and some internal organs
SS is further divided into:
- CREST:
    - Calcinosis   - Raynaud's phenomena
    - Esophageal dysmotility - Sclerodactyly   - Telangiectasia

Also associated with isolated pulmonary hypertension.
- Diffuse SS
    - Skin thickening involves both extremities and trunk.
    - Rapid onset after Raynaud's phenomena
    - Pulmonary fibrosis common

Identify life-threatening complications of SS
- Congestive heart failure (CHF)   - Pulmonary embolism   - Pericarditis
- Cardiac tamponade   - Arrhythmias

Treat ischemic digits with IV prostaglandins (prostacyclin)
It is important to address this problem emergently to avoid or reduce the loss of digits.

Identify pts with renal crisis and treat with ACE inhibitors
Renal crisis is defined as acute oliguric renal failure with malignant hypertension.
Risk factors include pregnancy, steroid use, and diffuse disease.
Educate pt early in disease about close monitoring of blood pressure and prophylactic use of ACE inhibitors to avoid renal crisis.

Educate all pts about disease progression and prognosis
Immunizations such as influenzae and pneumococcal

Treat symptoms of SS
Treatment aimed at symptom relief:
- Skin moisturizers for dryness   - Antihistamines for pruritus
- BP control with ACE inhibitors   - Proton pump inhibitor for reflux
- Anti-inflammatories like NSAIDs and COX-2 inhibitors for arthritis
- Calcium channel blockers (nifedipine) for Raynaud's
- Smoking cessation and avoidance of cold temperatures

Treat pulmonary hypertension with home oxygen and IV epoprostenol
Management of CHF is also an important component of therapy.
IV epoprostenol (improves exercise capacity)
Consider use of anticoagulation.

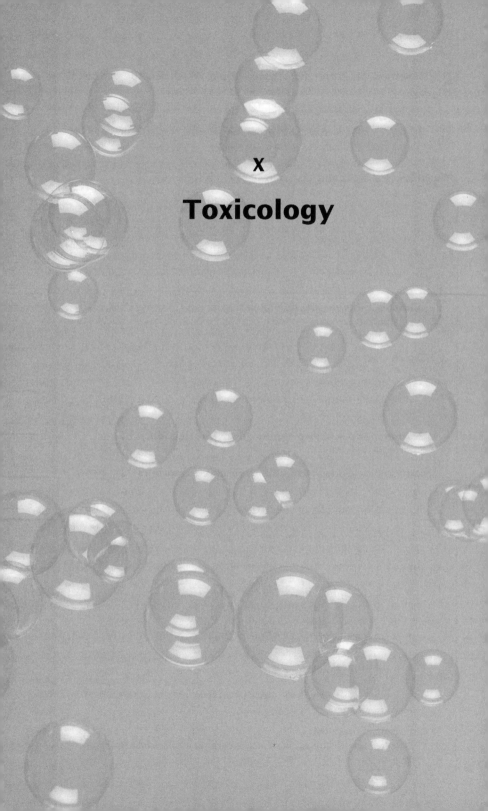

X

Toxicology

S   **How much does the pt normally drink? When was the pt's last drink?**
This information can aid in anticipation and management of withdrawal symptoms.
The alcohol-intoxicated pt generally may be unable to give a clear history.
- Family members, friends, and close contacts should be called to obtain information focusing on any coexisting medical problems, any history of trauma, last known drink, etc.

O   **Note vital signs and assess level of consciousness**
Tachycardia and fever can be signs of onset of delirium tremens.
A Glasgow Coma Score of less than 8 is an indication that intubation may be necessary.

Examine for signs of advanced or chronic liver disease

- Spider angiomata	- Caput medusae	- Palmar erythema
- Ascites	- Hepatomegaly	- Umbilical hernia
- Testicular atrophy	- Bilateral parotid swelling	- Peripheral neuropathy
- Prolonged PT, PTT	- Hypoalbuminemia	

Examine for evidence of GI bleeding
Hypotension, tachycardia, orthostatic BPs and pulse, decreasing hemoglobin and hematocrit on serial CBCs, and heme-positive stool

Check a serum alcohol level
A low level may indicate withdrawal or that another substance is responsible for the intoxication.
A serum alcohol level of greater than 400 mg/dL (0.4 gram%) is a risk of death and may require urgent hemodialysis.

Examine for possibility of other drug intoxication
Check urine and serum toxicology screen for any evidence of coexisting drugs.

Examine for evidence of other neurologic disorders
Seizure disorder, meningitis, head injury

Examine for glucose or electrolyte abnormalities
Pt is at increased risk for hypoglycemia if malnourished.
Low Mg, K, Phos are also common.
An anion gap acidosis or an elevated serum osmolality may indicate intoxication with methanol, ethylene glycol, or isopropanol. Ingestion of any of these substances may be fatal.
- Alcohol dehydrogenase in the liver converts ethanol to acetaldehyde. When this same chemical operation is performed on methanol, it is converted to formaldehyde.
- If ingestion of any of these substances is suspected, levels must be checked directly.

A   **Alcohol intoxication**
Alcohol is a central nervous system (CNS) depressant. Early effects include depression of inhibitions and later effects impair motor function, consciousness, and, at maximal concentrations, respiratory drive.

Differential diagnosis
CNS depressant drug intoxication such as barbiturates, benzodiazepines, or opioids
Pts may be intoxicated by more than one substance at once.

Consider intoxication with methanol, isopropyl alcohol, or ethylene glycol because chronic alcoholics may ingest these substances to attempt intoxication. Also consider infectious, neurologic, or psychiatric etiologies.

P **Monitor mental status**
Take aspiration precautions in case pt develops withdrawal seizures.
Consider intubation to protect airway.

Consider head CT for mental status changes or appearance of focal exam findings neurologic deficits
Optimize nutritional status by replacing magnesium, potassium, phosphorus, thiamine, and folate with an IV preparation known as a "banana bag"
Chronic alcohol abusers tend to be deficient in all of the above electrolytes and vitamins.
Chronic thiamine (vitamin B_1) deficiency can result in either Wernicke's or Korsakoff's encephalopathy.
  • Wernicke's is a triad of ophthalmoplegia, broad-based gait, and global confusion.
  • Korsakoff pts are demented to the point of confabulating.
Be sure to give thiamine before glucose to avoid precipitating Wernicke's encephalopathy.

If ingestion of ethylene glycol or methanol is suspected
Perform gastric lavage.
Give IV sodium bicarbonate to counteract the acid effects and alkalinize the urine to enhance elimination.
For ethylene glycol, activated charcoal may be given.
IV ethanol can be given to compete with these drugs for enzyme metabolism.

For potential isopropanol ingestion
Gastric lavage may be performed.
Charcoal and ethanol will be ineffective.
Consider hemodialysis.

Observe for and treat any signs of withdrawal
Changes in vital signs (fever, tachycardia, hypertension, tachypnea)
Anxiety
Tremor
Hallucinations: 48 to 72 hrs
Seizure activity: within 48 hrs of last drink
Delirium tremens: 48 hrs up to 2 wks
  • Treat with a short-acting benzodiazepine such as diazepam, lorazepam, or chlordiazepoxide. Chlordiazepoxide is the drug of choice for alcohol withdrawal provided that pts have normal liver function. If not, choose lorazepam.

Contact Social Services for appropriate rehabilitation referral

S **Does the pt give a history of drug use?**
If the pt is coherent, obtain the following information:
- Previous hospitalizations   • Length of drug abuse
- Drugs used and method of using them (e.g., smoking, snorting, intravenous)

Avoid aggravating an acutely intoxicated pt.

Contact family members or friends
Pts typically present altered and are unable to give a clear history.
The following information is important to obtain:

- Palpitations	- Chest pain	- Shortness of breath
- Headache	- Trauma	- Seizure activity
- History of suicide attempts	- Recent illness	- Change in mentation

O **Does the pt have VS suggestive of intoxication?**
- Tachycardia   - Hypertension   - Fever

Perform a thorough PE, with specific attention to the following
Gen: level of consciousness, anxiety, diaphoresis
HEENT: dilated pupils, dry mucous membranes, nasal sepatal perforation
Lungs: If the pt has used smokable crack–cocaine, look for pneumothorax.
Neuro: myoclonus, tremor, focal deficit, seizure
Skin: evidence of trauma

Review the results of the CBC with differential
Leukocytosis with left shift: consider infection. If seen, investigate the source.

Review urinalysis for signs of rhabdomyolysis
Look for moderate blood on dip with minimal RBCs on microscopy.
If suggestive, check CK level, electrolytes, phos and calcium, look for:
- Increased CK, BUN, creatinine, potassium, anion gap, and phosphorus
- Decreased calcium

Check serum and urine toxicology screen
Cocaine metabolites can be detected for up to 48 hrs or longer in chronic users.
Look for other stimulants (like amphetamines) or depressants (like alcohol).
- Their use increases the risk of cocaine toxicity.

Does the pt have an abnormal ECG?
Pt is at risk for ventricular arrhythmias or ischemia caused by cocaine-induced vasospasm. Consider checking troponin I or CK levels.

Consider taking a CXR
Pt is at risk for dissecting aortic aneurysm (chest pain radiating to back with widened mediastinum on CXR), cardiomegaly, or bilateral infiltrates.

Consider taking a head CT scan
Cocaine use is associated with acute cerebrovascular accidents.

A **Cocaine intoxication**
Cocaine is derived from the coca plant. It is an alkaloid that can be taken orally, nasally, intravenously, or smoked. It is a stimulant producing a wide range of symptoms, such as euphoria, tremor, agitation, headache, nausea, fever, and hypertension.
Cocaine overdose produces all of the above symptoms plus lethargy, hyperactive deep tendon reflexes (DTRs), seizures, hyperthermia, and incontinence. It also causes

severe vasoconstriction, which can cause vascular events like myocardial infarction (MI) and stroke. More severe manifestations are coma, loss of DTRs, flaccid paralysis, pulmonary edema, and sudden death from arrhythmia, stroke, MI, etc.

Chronic cocaine use can produce addiction, paranoia, and hallucinations.

Cocaine withdrawal can occur as soon as 15 minutes after last use and manifests as an inability to stay awake, excessive hunger, and paranoia.

Differential diagnosis

First consider co-ingestion of cocaine with other drugs, which is common:

- Alcohol, heroin (speedball), amphetamines, marijuana, etc.

Also consider other intoxications:

      - LSD   - Ecstasy   - Methamphetamines

A differential diagnosis depends on the manifestations your pt has, ranging from altered mental status to chest pain to anxiety and paranoia.

- Schizophrenia	- Anxiety	- Bipolar	- Delirium
- Dementia	disorder	disorder	- Uremia
- Lupus cerebritis	- Meningitis	- Encephalitis	- Neurosyphilis
- Stroke	- Diabetic ketoacidosis		

P Identify potentially life-threatening complications
Admit pt to a monitored bed and give supportive care

Cocaine overdose is a medical emergency, and interventions such as intubation may be necessary and the need for them should be monitored closely.

If pt is having an acute seizure, give a benzodiazepine IV

IV diazepam, approximately 2–10 mg/dose

If the seizure persists (> 10 min), give phenobarbital or phenytoin

Seizures lasting longer than 10 min should be treated as status epilepticus (see Seizure, p. 10).

If MI occurs, treat appropriately but avoid β-blockers

See Acute Coronary Syndrome, p. 34.

β-blockers are avoided because cocaine causes sympathetic stimulation including alpha (vasoconstrictive) effects, which will be unopposed with β blockade, leading to worse infarction as a result of vasospasm.

If arrhythmia occurs, identify and treat appropriately
If intracranial hemorrhage (cerebrovascular accident or subacute hemorrhage) occurs, transfer pt to the ICU and notify Neurosurgery

(See Cerebrovascular accident, p. 9)

Look for rhabdomyolysis and treat with fluid resuscitation

Check electrolytes and correct any abnormalities.

Consider renal consultation if renal function does not improve.

If pt is hyperthermic, consider neuroleptic malignant syndrome

Consider cooling measures, supportive care, bromocriptine, and dantrolene.

Chronic cocaine abuse requires a multidisciplinary approach

A social worker, psychiatrist, and a primary internist may all be needed for rehabilitation.

There are no medications effective for detoxification.

Cocaine withdrawal requires supportive care

Agitation may be controlled with IV or po benzodiazepines.

Appendix A Anemia: RBC morphology		
SIZE	**DESCRIPTION**	**ETIOLOGY**
Anisocytosis	Abnormal size variation	Any severe anemia
Macrocytes	Large Cells (MCV > 100)	Megaloblastic anemia, liver disease, hemolysis, liver disease, hypothyroid
Microcytes	Small Cells (MCV < 80)	Iron deficiency, sideroblastic anemia, thalassemia, lead poisoning
SHAPE	**DESCRIPTION**	**ETIOLOGY**
Acanthocytes	Small cells with thorn-like projections	Hereditary or post-splenectomy
Burr cells	Indented, shriveled cells	Hemolysis, uremia, DIC
Ovalocytes	Oval-shaped cells	Hereditary, iron deficiency
Poikilocytosis	Abnormal shape variation	Any severe anemia
Schistocytes	Fragmented cells	Intravascular hemolysis, post splenectomy
Sickle cells	Twisted crescent shape	Sickle cell
Spherocytes	Sphere-shaped cells	Hereditary, extravascular hemolysis, transfusion
Stomatocytes	Slit-like center (vs normally round center)	Hemolysis, thalassemia, burns, SLE, lead poisoning, liver disease
Target cells	Dark center in the middle of the normally clear center of the cell	Liver disease, thalassemia, hemoglobinopathy
Teardrop cells	Teardrop-shaped cells	Myeloproliferative, thalassemia
INCLUSIONS	**DESCRIPTION**	**ETIOLOGY**
Basophilic stippling	Small, dark dots (lead, iron)	Hemolysis, lead poisoning, thalassemia
Heinz bodies	Dark inclusions (denatured hemoglobin)	G6PD with hemolysis, some hemoglobinopathies
Howell-Jolly bodies	Purple spheres (nuclear debris)	Hyposplenism, pernicious anemia, thalassemia
Nucleated RBC	Nuclei still present (young RBC)	Hemolysis, myeloproliferative disease like leukemia, polycythemia vera, marrow infiltration, multiple myeloma, any severe anemia
Pappenheimer bodies	Blue granules (iron)	Sideroblastic (iron-loading) anemias, post-splenectomy

Index

Reactive arthritis, 155
Red blood cell mass, 94
Red cell distribution width, 90–91
Reiter's arthritis, 154
Renal failure
   acute, 70–71
   chronic, 72–73
Reticulocyte count, 91
Rhabdomyolysis, 168, 169
Rheumatoid arthritis, 152–153
Rheumatoid factor, 153
Rifampin, 21
Right upper quadrant pain, 54–55

S
Schober's test, 146
Sclerosis, systemic, 162–163
Seizures, 10–11
   vs. syncope, 6
Septic arthritis, 148, 149, 155
Seronegative spondyloarthropathy, 154–155
Sinus rhythm with premature beats, 43
Sinus tachycardia, 43
Sinusitis, 3
Sodium
   fractional excretion of, 71
   urinary, 78, 80
Solitary pulmonary nodule, 26–27
Spondyloarthropathy, seronegative, 154–155
Statins, 143
Stool, 62, 64
Straight-leg raise, 40, 146
Streptokinase, in pulmonary embolism, 23
Streptomycin, in tuberculosis, 21
Stroke, 8–9
Subarachnoid hemorrhage, 3
Superior vena cava syndrome, 108
Surgery, cardiac evaluation for, 46–47
Syncope, 6–7
Systemic lupus erythematosus, 158–159
Systemic sclerosis, 162–163
Systolic murmur, 38–39

T
Takayasu arteritis, 161
Tamponade, 44, 45
Temporal arteritis, 161
Tension headache, 2, 3
Tension pneumothorax, 31
Thiamine, 5, 167
Thrombocytopenia, 92–93
Thrombolytic therapy
   in pulmonary embolism, 23
   in stroke, 9

Thyroid hormones
   deficiency of, 4, 130
   excess of, 132–133
Thyroid storm, 4, 133
Thyroidectomy, 133
Thyroiditis, 131, 133
Tilt table testing, 7
Tissue plasminogen activator, in stroke, 9
Transfusion, platelet, 93
Tricuspid regurgitation, 39
Tricuspid stenosis, 40
Trigeminal neuralgia, 3
Trimethoprim-sulfamethoxazole, in urinary tract infection, 87
Troponin I, 34
Tuberculin skin test, 20–21
Tuberculosis, 20–21, 45
Tumor lysis syndrome, 84, 101

U
Ultrasound
   in breast mass, 105
   in deep vein thrombosis, 98
   of kidneys, 72
   in prostate cancer, 112
Uric acid, 100, 151
Urinary tract infection, 86–87
Urine
   blood in, 76–77
   potassium in, 85
   protein in, 74, 75
   sodium in, 78, 80
Urokinase, in pulmonary embolism, 23

V
Valsalva maneuver, murmur with, 38
Vasculitis, 160–161
Ventilation-perfusion scan, in pulmonary embolism, 22
Verapamil, in atrial fibrillation, 43
Vertebrobasilar insufficiency, 12
Vertigo, 12–13
Vitamin K deficiency, 97
Vomiting, bleeding with, 64

W
Warfarin, in deep vein thrombosis, 99
Water deficit, 81
Wegener's syndrome, 161
Wernicke-Korsakoff syndrome, 5, 167
Westermark sign, 22
Wilson's disease, 57, 60

Z
Zollinger-Ellison syndrome, 50